The Art of Hypnosis

Mastering Basic Techniques

Third Edition

Part I of Diversified Client-Centered Hypnosis

(based on the teachings of Charles Tebbetts)

C. Roy Hunter, M.S., FAPHP

Crown House Publishing Limited

www.crownhouse.co.uk

www.crownhousepubishing.com

Crown House Publishing Ltd
Crown Buildings, Bancyfelin, Carmarthen, Wales, SA33 5ND, UK
www.crownhouse.co.uk

and

Crown House Publishing Company LLC
6 Trowbridge Drive, Suite 5, Bethel, CT 06801, USA
www.crownhousepublishing.com

British Library of Cataloguing-in-Publication Data
A catalogue entry for this book is available
from the British Library.

Print ISBN 978-184590439-5
Mobi ISBN 978-184590448-7
ePub ISBN 978-184590449-4

LCCN 2010921870

Previously published by Kendall/Hunt Publishing Company
under ISBN: 9780757511011

Printed and bound in the UK by
Gomer Press, Llandysul, Ceredigion

Dedication and Acknowledgements

This book is dedicated to the many thousands of people devoting their careers to help empower their clients through the art of hypnosis, and to all who believe in the benefits of hypnosis to facilitate positive change.

I owe a debt of gratitude beyond words to my late mentor and friend, Charles Tebbetts, for his guidance and priceless encouragement – not only for my work as a hypnotherapist, but also for my teaching professional hypnotherapy. I also wish to thank Dr. Dwight Damon for encouraging me to write this book. Special recognition and appreciation is also in order for Jonathan Chang, M.D., who valued this book enough to take time out of his busy schedule and contribute the artwork for the first edition.

And finally, my deepest gratitude goes to Jo-Anne, my wife, for her willingness to share so many hours of my time with all of you who read this book. Her love and support helped make this book a reality, and she well deserves to share my success.

Roy Hunter
Thanksgiving Day, 1993

Postscript: As the second decade of the new millennium dawns, I wish to give thanks to all the professionals who use and endorse previous versions of this book. My gratitude also goes to the many hypnosis instructors who recommend this text as required reading for their students, and to all those responsible for selling out my previous editions so quickly. Also, as some have requested, this third edition contains a glossary. Since I made only minor changes to the 2010 version published by Crown House Publishing, this is still the third edition.

Table of Contents

Preface

by Ormond McGill, Ph.D.

It would be fun to say this is a spooky and mysterious book; but that would not be true, as it is a highly informative and scientific test about an *important* subject that is daily gaining increasing recognition – and is of personal value to everyone: *HYPNOTHERAPY.*

This book is written by a man who is an expert in this field, and was specially selected to carry on the work of a "grand master of hypnotherapy," the late beloved and esteemed Charles Tebbetts.

Charles Tebbetts was a master teacher and contributor to the art/ science of hypnosis; and his protégé, Roy Hunter, is remarkably skilled to carry on his work, of which this book is positive proof.

Today hypnosis is no longer shrouded in shadows, but in the bright light of understanding it is recognized as a remarkable means of controlling man's greatest gift: *the human mind.*

Mind is a process of producing thoughts, and when under the owner's perfect control it can lead to joyful living and heights of genius. The classic quote says: *"As a man thinkest in his heart, so is he."*

Roy Hunter has wonderfully contributed to the profession of hypnotherapy in this book, which in clear language all can easily comprehend; he explains what hypnosis is, how to induce it, and how to use this unique state of mind for benefit in countless ways.

Roy Hunter brings the understanding and practical use of hypnosis up-to-date. Just check the contents and you will instantly know the value of the book you hold in your hands.

Read it from cover to cover. You will not only learn about the *Art of Hypnotherapy* via the Charles Tebbetts methodology; you will also learn how to avoid being mastered by your mind, and instead will learn how to become a Mastermind.

Ormond McGill, Ph.D.
Palo Alto, CA
April 27, 1996

Introduction

by Conrad Adams, Ph.D.

Every profession has within its circle a few who are considered to be the master teachers. These dedicated teachers take the knowledge they have accumulated, digest it, add to it, refine it and then graciously pass along the end result through their daily work and mentoring activities. Their goal is to improve upon their chosen profession. Their challenge is to become an integral part of the evolution and growth of their discipline so that it impacts upon the world in the most positive way possible. These masters refuse to place themselves above those they serve. Instead, they give of themselves wholeheartedly by sharing their knowledge and promoting the well being of those they serve and teach. In doing so they become the examples to follow and the profession they serve is enriched. Roy Hunter is such a master teacher.

One of the most rewarding experiences a teacher can have is to observe a student take what has been learned, expand upon it, experiment with it, succeed with it and then passionately teach it to others so that they, too, may reap rewards from the knowledge. To see this occur is an affirmation that the knowledge taught is useful, important and appreciated.

Roy Hunter's mentor, Charles Tebbetts (honored by his peers as a master trainer of hypnotherapy) certainly enjoyed that rewarding experience when he asked his protégé to teach for him. And he certainly made a wise decision in doing so. That opportunity to teach for Charles Tebbetts inspired Roy Hunter and allowed him to evolve into the mentor he is today. If Charles Tebbetts were still with us today, he would undoubtedly be very proud of Roy Hunter for what he has done and continues to do by promoting quality education for the profession of hypnotherapy.

My mentor and friend, Dr. E. Arthur Winkler, Founder and President of St. John's University, often spoke highly of Roy Hunter and made references to his work as well as his integrity, professionalism and dedication to the spiritual aspects of the art and science of hypnotherapy. Since meeting Roy Hunter I have experienced first hand these qualities and the effectiveness of his teaching style at conferences and other workshops. His reputation sets an example for others in our profession to follow.

As I read *The Art of Hypnosis* I became amazed at the vast amount of subject material that has been compressed into the pages of one book. Roy Hunter starts with the very fundamentals of hypnosis and then takes the reader on an expansive journey into the fascinating art and science of hypnotherapy and how to use it effectively to promote health and wellness.

The author uses clear and precise language in a step-by-step approach to introduce the reader to the many facets of hypnotic technique. He incorporates a wide range of topics that offer an excellent overview of hypnosis for both the beginning practitioner and seasoned professional alike. *The Art of Hypnosis* is an easy read full of valuable information to be utilized for optimum results with clients.

Change is inevitable. Society is certainly experiencing change today seemingly more rapidly than at any other time in mankind's history. Hypnotherapy is a part of that change. There is a trend now for wider acceptance of hypnotherapy by medical professionals who are turning to its use as an adjunct to traditional healthcare modalities. Today's progressive hospitals are adjusting to this trend by creating separate departments of complementary medicine that incorporate the use of hypnotherapy.

If we are to adjust to this ever-constant and rapid change, we must be prepared to make mental changes quickly and efficiently. *The Art of Hypnosis* introduces its reader to valuable tools to be used to help evolve through these changes. It offers both self-hypnosis techniques and hypnotherapist directed techniques to facilitate subconscious change that is in agreement with the client's conscious desires. The end result is most often permanent and desirable behavioral change.

Few books on the subject of hypnosis cover such a wide spectrum of topics on the fundamentals of hypnotherapy. It is informative, enlightening, practical and constructive. Every hypnotherapist's personal library should include a copy of *The Art of Hypnosis*. It is a required text for students of Alpha University who are learning the art and science of hypnotherapy.

Conrad Adams, Ph.D.
Founder & Academic Dean
Alpha University
February, 2010

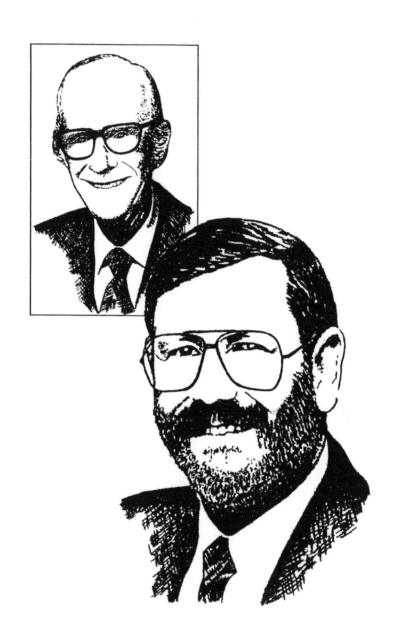

Chapter 1

Overview

Charles Tebbetts, a living legend, demonstrated what he taught:

> *"All hypnosis is self-hypnosis. If you follow my simple instructions, no power on earth outside yourself can keep you from being hypnotized ..."*

Following these words, countless numbers of people proceeded to experience what Mr. Tebbetts called Miracles on Demand. Many lives were profoundly improved; and those of us who were privileged to study hypnotherapy directly under the "grand master" of hypnosis found our lives forever touched.

The Purpose of This Book

What is it about the Charles Tebbetts Hypnotism Training Course that inspires me to continue teaching the Tebbetts methodology when there are so many other good training courses available today? The answer is contained within these pages.

Before using hypnosis to help people, we must first master basic techniques. The purpose of this book is to help you learn the art of hypnosis by mastering the same legendary basic techniques taught by the late "grand master" himself, enhanced and modified by my experience and presented in my style – *as taught to my own students at Tacoma Community College since 1987.* Also, since this author finds it easier to communicate in the first-person format, the reader will notice that I do so frequently throughout this book. (My former mentor did likewise.)

Several hypnotherapists urged me to write this book originally because *Miracles on Demand* (written by Charles Tebbetts) went out of print in October, 1993. Charlie's work MUST be preserved; and events of the late 1980s and early 1990s made me the best candidate for this. In 1993, Dr. Dwight Damon (President of the National Guild of Hypnotists) agreed, and encouraged me to write it, and you have the third version of the result in your hands.

The Charles Tebbetts Hypnotism Training Course was originally taught in three parts, as is my college course. The 500+ page work to back it up required two texts, and this is the first. My original title was: *The Art of Hypnosis: The Charles Tebbetts Methodology as Taught by Roy Hunter.* I changed the title three times since.

Furthermore, as the true artist is more interested in how to *master* an art instead of understanding why it works, this book strays from the usual academic writing style of typical textbooks. Rather than making this look like just another research paper, I use my own writing style – presenting the techniques of Charles Tebbetts just as I teach them to my own students.

Included are opinions of my former teacher and mentor as well as my own opinions, with updates of his work resulting from my own *experience* rather than on scientific research alone. Also, I write in simple language, just as my teacher taught in a friendly, easy-to-understand style. I hope you'll find this to be a fresh, new approach to learning.

With every class I begin at Tacoma, I present a brief overview of the entire course and preface my remarks with some words about my former mentor; so I'll do likewise here.

Who was Charles Tebbetts?

Dr. John C. Hughes, Research Editor of the National Guild of Hypnotist's international publication entitled *The Journal of Hypnotism*, referred to Charles Tebbetts as one of the "grand masters" of hypnosis. In 1990 he was honored and inducted into the International Hypnosis Hall of Fame for lifetime achievement. Charles Francis, author of *Counseling Hypnotherapy*, states that Mr. Tebbetts "… was generally considered the oldest and most experienced hypnotherapist in the world" (p. 152) prior to his passing. Additionally, he was respected from coast to coast by members of all the large professional hypnotherapy associations, where he frequently presented his legendary *parts therapy* techniques.

With over six decades' experience in the art of hypnotism, Mr. Tebbetts – who mastered many rapid-change client-centered techniques – taught that *all hypnosis is self-hypnosis*. In fact, Benjamin Franklin reached this same conclusion in the late 1700s, observing that Dr. Anton Mesmer's patients were responding to Mesmer's magnetism because of what was taking place in their own imaginations rather than because of any "mystical" power that Mesmer had. In other words, if the power resided in the minds of Mesmer's patients, then he was only facilitating their own self-mesmerism! (I'll discuss this further in the history chapter.) Yet instead of accepting this fact, most people since Mesmer still prefer to believe that the hypnotist has some "power" over others … and there are a few even today who attempt to use hypnosis to trick people into giving up their power.

In reality, the hypnotist is only a practitioner skilled in the art of guided self-hypnosis, as the individual creates his or her own trance state by following instructions of the artist. Yet even now, many researchers who are seriously interested in hypnotism still tend to research it only as a "science" rather than recognizing it as an art.

Mr. Tebbetts believed that if the hypnotist really mastered hypnotism as an *art*, this would diminish the likelihood of client resistance. Not only did he often have profound results with clients, he became a master teacher who taught hypnotherapy in a way that made him a living legend prior to his passing.

One of the most unique professional qualities about the Charles Tebbetts I knew was the way he endeavored to *make things simple.* He felt this was the best way to use hypnosis; and so do I, as should be evidenced by this book.

3

He believed that a client-centered therapist mastering a variety of simple techniques could be far more effective than the scholar of hypnosis who fails to create rapport with the client even though he/she might have a wealth of knowledge about scientific research in various applications of hypnosis.

While science tends to walk with a microscope, most clients are more interested in results than in getting bogged down with labels and scientific *whys*, etc. Thus, Mr. Tebbetts believed that some of the most simple concepts, once communicated effectively to the subconscious, could bring about some of the most profound changes in people's lives. He proved this time after time in his class at Edmonds, Washington, with the way he demonstrated his mastership of the art of hypnosis.

Originally Charles Tebbetts became interested in hypnosis while playing in a band and observing a stage hypnotist; and he eventually performed the show himself when the hypnotist was unable to do so. This began a lifetime career of hypnosis, interwoven with other careers until he reached middle age. After studying hypnotherapy seriously in Southern California with Gil Boyne, he set up a full-time practice. Eventually he moved to Edmonds, Washington, where he taught professional hypnotism until the end of 1991. In 1987 he decided to expand his hypnotism training course to another city by asking me to teach it under his supervision. Then, in 1992, he moved to Arkansas where he spent most of his final months.

His passing took place among his peers in August that same year, at the annual convention of the National Guild of Hypnotists. Mr. Tebbetts was scheduled to present a workshop on his legendary *parts therapy* techniques, but he suffered a heart attack. He asked me to present in his behalf, and then passed on while I was quoting from his writings during his workshop. This was a very emotional experience for me; and I consider it an honor that my mentor asked me to continue his teachings.

By providing a written record of how I both utilize and teach the rapid change techniques of Charles Tebbetts, as enhanced through my own professional experience, it is my hope to preserve my late mentor's teachings through the 21st century and beyond. Originally I assumed that my entire course would go into one book divided into three parts – but because of the length of this first book on *mastering basic techniques*, it seemed appropriate to publish this first volume as a separate text for the new student of hypnosis.

Now let me summarize the objectives of my entire course, which I now call *Diversified Client-Centered Hypnosis*, based on the course I originally started teaching at Tacoma Community College in 1987.

Part I: Learning the Art of Basic Hypnosis

The primary objective is to help the student of hypnosis to *master basic skills and knowledge* in the art of hypnosis. We must learn to walk before we can learn how to run and do other exercises; and the same is true with hypnosis. One must master the *ART OF HYPNOSIS* before effectively using hypnotic techniques to help people change habits and achieve goals – hence the title for this book.

Basic hypnotic techniques must be learned and mastered before learning the effective use of hypnotherapy techniques, because of a simple truth. *All hypnotherapy employs the use of hypnosis; but not all hypnosis is hypnotherapy.*

The BASIC course, as taught by Charles Tebbetts in the 1980s, was simplified and easy to learn. He incorporated suggestibility tests to help prepare a client for hypnosis. He categorized all hypnotic inductions into six basic induction types, and taught enough induction techniques to incorporate all six types.

We broke into pairs to practice all the basic techniques Tebbetts taught in the classroom, while our teacher observed and supervised the practice sessions.

After learning inductions, the hypnosis student then learned several deepening techniques as well as several hypnotic "convincers" to help the client believe in the hypnotic experience. We again broke into pairs to practice deepening techniques as well as the "convincers" that Tebbetts taught.

Next, the student now learned how to give effective non-therapeutic post-hypnotic suggestion as further evidence to the client that he/she really did experience hypnosis, and we learned how to construct more effective suggestions. Also included was a class on self-hypnosis.

My mentor's course included his opinions and concepts based on several decades of experience, woven throughout the course. I added these where appropriate, and devoted Chapter 11 of this book exclusively to some of the basic ones Charles Tebbetts emphasized. He only briefly discussed hypnosis history, encouraging us to study on our own; but I included a lengthy history chapter, and discuss it in my own basic hypnosis class.

Since an *art must be experienced* in order to be learned, Charlie emphasized practice to help develop confidence and competence. I concur, so I encourage the reader of this book to seek actual "hands on" training in hypnosis rather than simply relying on books alone for learning and mastering the art of hypnosis, ESPECIALLY if there is any intention of using hypnosis for therapeutic purposes.

In addition to adding some historical background on hypnosis in my classroom, I discuss ethics, legalities and potential dangers – and have also included them in this book. I also added the important "hypnotic formula" to the very first class.

My mentor was a pioneer, so his course is now updated and combined with some of my own material. We all must grow, but I still endeavor to preserve the integrity of his methodology. My basic course still resembles his "101" course greatly, and I still endeavor to keep it simple.

While Charles Tebbetts was still living, I initiated frequent communication to discuss my updates, and to solicit approval on the added material where necessary. He deserved this courtesy since my course was based on his client-centered teachings. My students seem satisfied with the results; I trust that you will be as well.

Part II: *Learning the Art of Hypnotherapy*

Once you learn how to walk with the basic hypnosis techniques, what next?

At Tacoma Community College, Part II attempts to answer that question. As with the Basic quarter, emphasis is more on *"how to"* rather than on scientific or academic documentation. Since client results speak louder than words, client results are threaded throughout my second book based on The Charles Tebbetts Hypnotism Training Course – including some discussions of actual case histories on record which he facilitated. It is entitled: *The Art of Hypnotherapy.*

Client-centered hypnotherapy means much more to one who *first* masters a variety of basic hypnosis techniques. My former mentor always said, *"Deal with what emerges!"* Sometimes what emerges is a client who resists basic hypnotic techniques; therefore it is essential to fit the technique to the client rather than trying to fit the client to the technique. So with that in mind, Mr. Tebbetts taught and used a variety of techniques throughout his career, and taught me to do likewise.

The objective of what I once called the "intermediate segment" at Tacoma Community College is to teach the hypnotherapy student how to apply those techniques learned in the basic segment for habit control, general self-improvement, and personal motivation. I also want my students to learn how to help their clients discover and release any inhibitions or subconscious "blocks" preventing them from reaching a goal. My stated mission statement is to *help people attain their ideal empowerment;* and I teach my students to do likewise. Part II is now called: *Learning the Art of Hypnotherapy.*

The student first learns a foundation of four main steps to achieving successful hypnotherapy (summarized in the last chapter of this book). These steps form a foundation for all hypnotherapy techniques learned even beyond the class.

Included in *"Intermediate"* is information I teach on the *benefits approach* – which was added to my first class with my mentor's consent, who was my course sponsor while he lived (as well as my friend). Charles Tebbetts openly admitted that any hypnotic technique which helped a client overcome a problem or obtain a goal was worthy of professional consideration, provided it was not harmful or dangerous to the client; so he was quite willing to let me teach this somewhat original but effective approach. I've added an important class on anchors and triggers, because they relate directly to habit control.

Charlie's effective techniques help the subconscious to disclose the cause(s) of resistance to change, so that the client can be empowered to release the cause(s). Hypnotic regression therapy is explored in depth for a number of weeks, with emphasis on minimizing the risk of false memories. The hypnotherapist learns how to facilitate client abreactions during a hypnotic regression, how to avoid pitfalls such as unwisely "leading" the client during a regression, and how to use a variety of techniques to take a client back to the original cause of a problem ... and more.

This *cannot* be learned adequately in one weekend!

Part III: Advanced Hypnotherapy Techniques

This class takes a closer look at just how hypnotherapy goes beyond simple motivation. Actual case histories are summarized for further examination of the Tebbetts techniques, and we explore other techniques as well. I wove some into *The Art of Hypnotherapy* instead of writing a third text.

The rapid change techniques of Charles Tebbetts include his legendary *parts therapy* (also called "ego states" therapy), as well as other client-centered methods that help facilitate subconscious change. Students see some videotapes of actual therapy sessions facilitated by Mr. Tebbetts, showing how the "grand master" helped people change their lives.

My *"Advanced Hypnotherapy"* class at the college provides the student an exposure to the use of a variety of hypnotherapy techniques for more specialized areas and/or more serious problems as well, such as those that might require a medical referral. There are videos showing Mr. Tebbetts in action, revealing how he utilized his own techniques for some of these, such as helping an alcoholic victim of epilepsy overcome both of those problems. The actual therapy script of this particular case, along with a testimonial, is included in my next book.

A few advanced techniques are touched on during Part III, and some are included in *The Art of Hypnotherapy*; but this class is always open to change, as I bring in guest presenters whenever possible. (Additionally, there are a few highly qualified instructors in other cities teaching my course in a similar manner, utilizing student materials and study guides in addition to my texts.)

I wish to give my students an opportunity for learning new techniques – including some that go beyond what either Charles Tebbetts taught or what I've developed and/or enhanced from his teachings over the years. With this in mind, the serious student of hypnotherapy is encouraged to grow beyond my books and follow the recommendations of several professional hypnosis associations: *pursue ongoing continuing education.*

In all of your pursuits to further your skills in the use of hypnotism, however, use only those techniques which benefit your clients – and then master them with both confidence and competence.

Now let's get started with the first book ...

Chapter 2

Hypnosis:
What IS It and Why Use It?

Hollywood shrouds hypnosis in mysticism, and it is way past time to take it out of the dark ages! It is not mind control, nor is the hypnotized person "under someone's power" as we are led to believe by the movies. Nor is it some dangerous scientific tool that should only be used by physicians or people with advanced academic degrees – because degrees do not guarantee ethics.

However, if we are going to seriously consider mastering the art of hypnosis, we need to know *what* it is, what its main *ingredients* are, and *why* we should use it.

Before examining what it is, let's talk about its benefits.

Why Use Hypnosis?

Have you ever tried to change a habit pattern, or become more self-motivated, only to find your subconscious mind resisting? The very fact that the subconscious can create such resistance to change is WHY we often need hypnotherapy.

In the very first chapter of his book, *Self-Hypnosis and Other Mind-Expanding Techniques* (third edition), Charles Tebbetts wrote:

> *Since the subconscious mind is our driving force, we always do what our subconscious believes. Since it will believe anything it is told, we*

11

> can reprogram it if we bypass the conscious mind and substitute new,
> constructive ideas for its existing negative ones. (p. 6)

My clients frequently ask me why they find themselves unable to accomplish seemingly simple goals and objectives through willpower. My response is to explain that acceptance of any new habit pattern requires subconscious cooperation, otherwise your conscious decision to make the desired change is undermined by your own subconscious belief in failure.

There is a basic law of the mind at work here: *whenever your conscious and subconscious are in conflict, your subconscious invariably wins!*

This is called the law of conflict. It can also be stated another way, *whenever imagination and logic are in conflict, imagination usually wins.*

This has been proven repeatedly: by smokers unable to stop without outside help, by dieters constantly going up and down with their weight, by outgoing people suddenly finding themselves petrified with fright when speaking in public, and by each of us as we wonder why things we want to change in life do not come easily.

People usually try to change their habits through willpower and/ or self-discipline. While they may convince themselves what the *logical* course of action is, they still *imagine* themselves doing what they subconsciously desire to do. For example, smokers trying to quit still *imagine* the taste or smell of cigarettes, or dieters *imagine* how good junk food would taste – and then wonder why they backslide into old habits.

Imagination does usually win out over logic – and since this is true, we must be motivated to change at a subconscious level in order to change a habit permanently. We could also put this another way: willpower does not have a very good track record with changing habits, but *hypnosis does!*

As hypnosis and/or self-hypnosis are both proving to be effective ways to facilitate change at a subconscious level, this has resulted in increasing interest in the benefits of hypnosis and self-hypnosis! This rapidly increasing interest in hypnosis has created a rapidly evolving profession with thousands of professionals dedicated to the beneficial uses of hypnosis: *the hypnotherapy profession.*

Subconscious Resistance to Change

All of our present habits, mannerisms, and thought patterns are the results of past subconscious "programming" from parents, teachers, peers, co-workers, television – a variety of sources.

This programming can either propel us into success against all odds – or keep us from it in spite of our best efforts. In order to succeed, then, it becomes vitally important for us to learn how to gain and maintain control of our own subconscious programming.

Virtually all of us experience the difficulty of changing a habit pattern at one time or another. Once your subconscious learns something, it tends to *resist change;* and the more you try to force the change, the greater the resistance.

The subconscious acts like a child who resents force and rebels. Yet people spend countless megabucks on various self-help books, smokers' treatments, various diet clinics, motivation programs, tapes, consultants, psychotherapists, and other professionals, seeking help to change old habits.

Logic works with the conscious mind, but imagination is the language of the subconscious. Hypnosis helps the subconscious by enhancing the ability to imagine ... yet *negative imagination* can defeat both positive thinking as well as the strongest logic!

For example, I have been told by numerous diet counselors that 97 percent of people who pay money to lose weight find it again in less than two years. In other words, *diets work on the body but not the mind;* and unless the subconscious is changed, willpower is only temporary.

"Old Tapes" Must Be Changed

In hypnotherapy, we refer to subconscious programming as "old tapes" since our minds retain everything. (Someday we might change that to "Old CDs" rather than tapes.)

Some old tapes are good. We may be programmed to stop automatically at a red light, brush our teeth every day, say "thank you" when appropriate and act according to certain social standards, etc. We accept these tapes without thinking about them. But we also accept other tapes such as "I have my father's temper," or "I'm lousy with math," or "All my relatives are overweight, because it runs in the family."

When the subconscious mind is full of negative program tapes, it's virtually impossible to stay in a positive frame of mind unless those tapes are changed on a subconscious level. The hypnotherapist who is skilled at the art of hypnosis can greatly enhance a client's ability to replace and rewrite old tapes, and to make profound changes in a positive way!

What is Hypnosis?

Hypnosis has been given so many definitions that I could write for hours with commentaries on all the various definitions I've encountered over the years. Even as the new millennium dawns, professionals are still unable to agree on an exact definition!

The Mosby Medical Encyclopedia (1992 edition) defines hypnosis as "a passive, trancelike state that resembles normal sleep during which perception and memory are changed, resulting in increased responsiveness to suggestion."

I prefer the way Charles Tebbetts defines hypnosis, and will quote from his second edition of *Miracles on Demand*:

> *There is no legal definition of hypnosis. Webster's dictionary describes it incorrectly as an artificially induced sleep, but it is actually a natural state of mind and induced normally in everyday living much more often than it is induced artificially. Every time we become engrossed in a novel or a motion picture, we are in a natural hypnotic trance. (pp. 211–212)*

Mr. Tebbetts went on in his book (and his class) to explain that hypnosis exhibits several identifying characteristics including: an extraordinary quality of mental, physical and emotional relaxation, a partial absence of the inhibitory process, or – as he so frequently said in class – a bypassing of the critical faculty of the mind. He also touches on the four states of mind, which I describe later in this chapter.

Dr. John C. Hughes, in his book, *Hypnosis: the Induction of Conviction* (pub. by National Guild of Hypnotists), says:

> *Hypnosis is one of the seven wonders of modern psychology. No one really knows what hypnosis is. But then no one knows what electricity is either. Yet that does not deter its usefulness. (p. 14)*

Dr. Hughes goes on to point out that Hippolyte Bernheim believed there was no hypnosis, only suggestion; and that Emile Coué, the father of autosuggestion, believed that there is no suggestion – only autosuggestion. Or, stated another way, we could consider that all hypnosis is *guided autosuggestion!*

The very word *hypnosis*, coined by an English physician in the 19th century, has given us an inaccurate picture for well over a century. It is derived from the Greek word *hypnos*, meaning sleep. But hypnosis is not a state of sleep. Rather, it is the same state of altered conscious awareness we enter daily when our brainwave activity slows down to a frequency called "alpha," which we pass through on the way to and from sleep. Many experts also refer to it as "altered consciousness" since the mind of a hypnotized person is still aware of what is taking place even though he/she may *appear* to be sleeping. (In fact, some clients are surprised at how aware they are during the hypnotic process – yet they still achieve benefits.)

I totally agree with the theory Charles Tebbetts taught: all hypnosis is self-hypnosis, so the hypnotherapist is more like a guide who facilitates the hypnotic process. Myron Teitelbaum, M.D., author of *Hypnosis Induction Technics* (spelling by Dr. Teitelbaum), came to the same conclusion – as is evidenced in the last two pages of Chapter 3:

> *The hypnotist is merely the guide who directs and leads the subject into the trance. (p. 18)*

To me, the most accurate way of defining hypnosis is to simply refer to it as *guided meditation*.

Since many of us enter a meditative or "trance" state while listening to music, watching television, listening to a good speaker or a good sermon at church, or even while reading a good book, you could say that the hypnotist does not even have to be a live person. So if hypnosis were ever outlawed, it would be virtually impossible to enforce, because we would have to stop the freedom of speech and freedom of press!

On the other hand, if all hypnosis is – as Charles Tebbetts firmly believed – really guided self-hypnosis, then that truly makes the hypnotist an *artist!*

Hypnosis = Altered Consciousness

I frequently explain hypnosis to a prospective client by asking a question such as, "When is the last time you cried real tears during a powerful movie? Even though your conscious mind knew you were sitting in a theater watching actors and actresses, your subconscious accepted them as real characters because you were in the state of hypnosis! And when I saw the movie *E.T.*, it seemed like everyone in the theater cried, including me."

Was I asleep when I saw *E.T.*? Not at all! Yet even though my conscious mind knew it was only a six-million dollar puppet, my subconscious accepted E.T. as a real character. Although I was literally hypnotized, I was very aware of what was happening in the movie – but soon became able to "tune out" the usually incessant coughing, straw-slurping and throat-clearing among theater audiences. Even though I was not in a sleep state, I was definitely in an altered state of consciousness. Other movies can have similar effects on us.

Even though the "critical faculty" can be bypassed when we get engrossed in the movie, that motion picture does *not* control us; it *only guides* us through its story. It could be said, then, that the movie is our hypnotist until the closing credits cross the screen.

The same is true when a person becomes the hypnotist. Because the conscious mind has relaxed, the subconscious mind becomes accessible, thus giving us expanded possibilities for change; however, the hypnotist does not control us. Rather, he/she only becomes our guide during the hypnotic experience. The actual power for change is within the mind of the person who enters the state of hypnosis.

Also, because hypnosis is not a "sleep" state but actually an altered state of consciousness, people frequently do not feel hypnotized the first time they go to a hypnotherapist. This is partly because of the fact that we all experience four different mental states daily. These states of mind can be measured by an E.E.G. (electroencephalograph).

According to Dr. Barbara B. Brown, author of *Stress and the Art of Biofeedback,* experts vary in their opinions on the exact range of alpha and theta waves. However, since this is meant to be a *How To* book for the art of hypnotherapy rather than a scientific or academic treatise, I will only briefly discuss the four basic mental states shown on the next page.

The Four States Of Mind

Brainwave patterns as measured by an E.E.G. machine

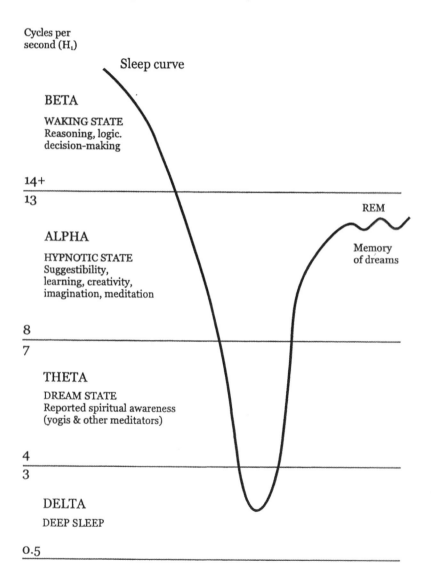

Cycles per
second (H₁)

Sleep curve

BETA

WAKING STATE
Reasoning, logic.
decision-making

14+

13

REM

ALPHA

HYPNOTIC STATE
Suggestibility,
learning, creativity,
imagination, meditation

Memory
of dreams

8

7

THETA

DREAM STATE
Reported spiritual awareness
(yogis & other meditators)

4

3

DELTA

DEEP SLEEP

0.5

The Four States of Mind

You are in the *beta* state for most of your waking hours. It's a good thing, too, since beta is like high gear – a good place for decision making, reasoning and logic. Brainwaves are above 13 cycles per second, often greatly higher, and may or may not be rhythmic.

As your brainwaves slow to between 8 and 13 cycles per second, you enter the *alpha* state of mind. The door between your conscious and subconscious minds is opened, and it becomes easier to access the memories and storage of new information. We may become mellow in this relaxed state; we are also more suggestible – and this is what Hollywood exploits in movies and stage hypnosis.

When you are guided into the alpha state of mind by another person or thing (whether a movie, CD, or person) you are technically hypnotized.

Below the two conscious states are *theta*, the dream state, and *delta*, which is deep sleep or total unconsciousness. Whether or not you remember your dreams, you must pass through theta on the way to and from delta. Likewise, you must pass through alpha on the way to and from sleep. You are in the same state of mind as hypnosis every day of your life! I've taught this for years, including it in a book in 1987.

Within a month after my self-hypnosis book hit the press, a psychologist specializing in study of brainwaves informed me that recent discoveries had indicated that the brain still produces alpha waves even when we are in a total conscious state of *beta* (simultaneous alpha and beta waves). At first that bothered me, creating a concern that I might have written incorrect data. Soon afterwards, I received further clarification that the subconscious mind usually stays in alpha – at walking speed – while the conscious mind jogs along in *beta*. Then, when we enter hypnosis (or meditation), both conscious and subconscious slow down to alpha – or walking speed – enhancing communication between both these parts of the mind.

Since opinions still vary, you are free to draw your own conclusions and/or do your own research or scientific investigations. What is important, however (if you intend to help people achieve their goals), is to master hypnosis as an art rather than as something that you do strictly from the intellectual mind. I both practice and teach hypnosis as an *art* rather than a science; so I will repeat and emphasize my own opinion with all who read this book: *hypnosis is an art* – and to master the art, you must *practice*.

Charles Tebbetts believed that there is no substitute for practice to develop confidence and competence; therefore my students must complete at least 24 practice sessions of non-therapeutic hypnosis during Part I of *Diversified Client-Centered Hypnosis* (formerly called Part I of the Charles Tebbetts Hypnotism Training Course). Much of this is done in a supervised setting in my classroom; and this book presents the actual techniques that my students learn and practice.

With clients I may or may not go into the explanation of the four states of mind, depending on the person I'm working with. Also, note that I always refer to people who see me in my office as *clients*.

Terminology for People in Hypnosis

What do you call people who are hypnotized? There are different words that can be used. Allow me to explain my views on when it is appropriate to use different terminology, starting with the word used most commonly:

Subjects

Subjects are people who are used in scientific experiments with hypnosis, or who allow themselves to become the willing "subjects" of unscientific experimenting by someone with minimal professional training (or sometimes none).

I have a strong personal preference to avoid most other uses of the word "subject" to identify one who is hypnotized; yet most books on hypnosis usually refer to the person who is being hypnotized as the *subject*. This negative word can be misleading as well as scary for some people, in that the very word itself implies that the person in hypnosis must *subject* himself/herself to the suggestions of the hypnotist. This word therefore incorrectly portrays hypnosis as a state of mind where one falls under the "power" of the hypnotist and is controlled by whatever suggestions are given. Thus, many still fear hypnosis today.

It is also my personal opinion that use of the word *subject* is also somewhat demeaning to a fee-paying person desiring the benefits of hypnosis for self-empowerment to achieve a goal. Throughout my entire book (with some exceptions in Chapter 3) I use the term *client*, which is (in my opinion) more dignified and respectful of the person in hypnosis. Even in references from Charles Tebbetts, I change the word "subject" except in direct quotes from one of his books.

Clients

Clients are people who (1) want their lives improved through the use of *non-medical* applications of hypnosis, or (2) are seeing a professional hypnotherapist (referred to as a "lay hypnotist" by some physicians and psychologists) for medical applications of hypnosis (such as pain management, etc.) with written consent of an examining physician – but done at the therapist's office rather than at the physician's clinic. This person is the client of the hypnotherapist, and the patient of his/her physician. It is considered that said hypnotherapist in this definition is one who is neither licensed to treat nor diagnose physical or mental illnesses.

Charles Tebbetts was training himself to use the word *client* more often in his latter years, as is evidenced by his frequent use of this word in *Miracles on Demand*.

Patients

Patients experiencing hypnosis are people who are (1) experiencing medical applications of hypnosis inside a hospital or medical clinic facilitated by a medical professional or by a hypnotherapist under medical supervision; (2) patients of a dental clinic hypnotized by either the dentist or a hypnotherapist at said clinic; or (3) a patient of any other licensed health care professional qualified to use hypnosis specifically as part of such health care treatment.

Participants

Participants are people experiencing non-medical applications of hypnosis done with a group of people at one time, such as when I work with a group of business people for stress management; with people hypnotized by students learning professional hypnosis; or with volunteers on stage experiencing stage hypnosis.

Ormond McGill referred to the volunteers in his stage hypnotism presentation as his *committee.* I also like his term for volunteers on stage, because it is respectful.

Remember, when you master the art of hypnosis, these are real people you are hypnotizing; and if you treat them with respect, you increase your probability of success.

Faith and Hypnosis are Closely Related

Back in 1983, Charles Tebbetts gave me a handout with the above title my very first evening at his class in Edmonds. Years later, he requested that I reproduce and provide, unedited, the same handout to my own students.

The material in this chapter subsection is reprinted just as written by Charles Tebbetts and, out of respect to my former teacher, nothing has been changed.

Belief

Belief plays an important part in hypnosis, and in the field of medicine as well.

Subconscious belief is the most powerful factor in successful living. It determines all behavior patterns. Yet belief systems are imposed upon our unwary minds during childhood before our critical factors are developed enough to reject harmful ideas that we would reject at a later period in our lives.

Our subconscious beliefs determine whether we will succeed or fail, be happy or unhappy, sick or well, and even if we will be dead or alive.

Self-confidence is belief in yourself.

Confidence is not competence. Most people lack competence in many fields, such as the ability to run the mile in record time, to lift 500 pounds of weight, or to win the figure skating championship – but they have confidence in themselves. They know that with practice they could learn to excel in any endeavor they choose.

When the subconscious mind is convinced, it starts to act. As hypnotherapists, our function is to convince the subconscious mind. While a person is in hypnosis, the more the conscious mind recedes, the more accessible the subconscious mind becomes – but consciousness does not disappear at any level.

Hypnosis is super concentration of the mind upon a single idea, and exclusion of all other thoughts.

*Hypnosis could be called **mono-ideaism**, in which the consciousness agreeably slows down to a single focus.*

The Three Psychological Principles of Suggestion

1. *The law of concentrated attention:* There is no action without a stimulus. While a person is in hypnosis he concentrates upon a single idea to the exclusion of all other thoughts, so when

he is told that his arm is so rigid that it will not bend, and no other thought is allowed to inhibit this idea, his arm will not bend because there is no stimulus.

2. *The law of reverse action:* This law is illustrated by the suggestion "The harder you try to bend your arm the more rigid it becomes" – and should be used with all tests to prove to the client that he is hypnotized.

3. *The law of dominant effect:* A stronger emotion will always overcome a weaker one. Emotional attachment to a suggestion makes it more effective. In a conflict between the conscious and the subconscious minds, the subconscious usually wins.

Hypnotic Formula: Components of Hypnosis

In the above chapter subsection, my mentor showed how faith and hypnosis are related. He discussed belief – which is one of several mental components of hypnosis.

There are other vital components, or what I sometimes call the ingredients of hypnosis. They include, besides belief, the ingredients of imagination, conviction and expectation. (An easy way to remember them is with the acronym B.I.C.E.)

These ingredients can either inhibit or insure the hypnotic state, depending on whether they are working positively or negatively with the client preparing for hypnosis. They also influence the outcome of a series of hypnotherapy sessions, whether the goal is motivation, habit control, or any other goal that relates to self-improvement.
Understanding these four ingredients is so important that I include this information in my very first class.

Charles Tebbetts examined all four of these ingredients of hypnosis at various times in his teaching, even thought not normally all at once. My own students have found that an early working knowledge of these vital ingredients becomes a very valuable asset in mastering the art of hypnosis. In simple terms, I call this the **Hypnotic Formula**. This is foundational for an understanding of how the subconscious works.

Imagination

Imagination enhances one's ability to be hypnotized, especially since imagination is the language of the subconscious – as is evidenced by the way we can all respond to something that is not real simply because we *imagine* it. I'll discuss this more in Chapter 4, showing how a simple investment of a few extra minutes before you hypnotize someone can help him/her to understand and appreciate the role of imagination in the hypnotic process, and is the *"holodeck" of the mind.*

If a person can easily imagine being hypnotized, he/she will find it much easier to enter the state of hypnosis. On the other hand, if one *imagines resisting*, guess what might be likely to happen! In other words, people who cannot imagine themselves being hypnotized by another person usually resist the hypnotic process.

Belief

Whatever a person *believes* will happen tends to come to pass if his/her own actions have anything to do with it.

If someone *believes* that you will successfully facilitate hypnosis, your probability of success is greatly increased. On the other hand, anyone who believes that he/she cannot be hypnotized – or believes that you cannot successfully facilitate hypnosis – will most likely resist.

Expectation and conviction

Expectation and conviction are like twins.

Those who are *convinced* that you can hypnotize them will most likely *expect* to be hypnotized – and your success is much more likely.

If one *expects* to succeed (or fail), and is totally *convinced* that it will happen, whatever expectation is believed and imagined will most likely be either the real result or the perceived result.

Mixing the Ingredients to Hypnosis

Belief + imagination + conviction + expectation = results. As mentioned earlier in this chapter, a good acronym to help you remember is BICE. (The order is not important, since belief often precedes imagination or vice versa.) Let's see how these ingredients mix together *during* the hypnosis session ...

Someone who imagines that he (or she) can indeed be hypnotized will influence both the belief and the expectation because of what takes place inside the imagination. This same person will find it much easier to imagine acting on the suggestions given, and will therefore have a far greater expectation of success. Without conviction, however, the person may or may not respond. Once the conviction is set, the probability of a successful outcome greatly increases unless that conviction is changed.

Imagination leads to belief (or vice versa), and these both lead to expectation and conviction regardless of the conscious desire. Additionally, this principle applies to habits as well as to the state of hypnosis. Note that the hypnotic formula can work in reverse for the skeptic who is convinced that hypnosis will not work.

Now let's examine how these ingredients relate to the client's success *after the session is over* ...

People who desire to stay on a diet but still *imagine* eating sweets will soon eat the sweets they *imagine* eating! A smoker desiring to quit will invariably have urges as long as he/she keeps *imagining* smoking. Worse, if that smoker keeps on fantasizing (or imagining) backsliding, he/she will almost always end up smoking once again.

How does belief influence long-term success? If the smoker firmly *believes* that he/she will never smoke again, the urges can be resisted because of the expectation; but this belief could be very easily influenced by the imagination. If he/she keeps on *imagining* the old fair-weather friend, those urges can persist even for years after smoking the last cigarette. Likewise, the weight-watchers who believe that they will find the weight they lose may end up heavier than before they started dieting.

If a client trying to break ANY bad habit *believes* that he/she will backslide into the old habit, the belief tends to manifest into reality even after an initial success. For this reason, it becomes important to help a client maintain all the ingredients of the hypnotic formula to help insure a longer lasting success.

Those clients who both imagine and believe in their ability to maintain long-term success will *expect* that success to be permanent ... and when your client combines these three ingredients with conviction, you will most likely have another satisfied client!

Let's review this in step-by-step order for the student of hypnotherapy.

The hypnotherapist must first help clients to *imagine* being hypnotized. Suggestibility tests (covered in Chapter 4) will help to accomplish this, as well as a proper discussion and explanation of hypnosis.
Secondly, clients must *believe* that they can be hypnotized, *and* that you are capable of facilitating that process. Then you must competently use hypnotherapy to help them *believe* that their goals are attainable.

Building on *imagination* and *belief*, then, your client must *expect* to be hypnotized and have a firm *conviction* that this will happen in order to insure success.

The hypnotist can use suggestions and guided imagery to help clients *imagine* successfully achieving their goals. Removal of any subconscious blocks of disbelief is handled through hypnotherapy rather than by suggestion alone (which is why the next book is a must for the professional). Finally, competent hypnotherapy can help the client release negative beliefs (at the cause) and build the expectation of success. This leads to a firm conviction that success is a reality ... empowering the client to make it so!

The greater the positive presence of these ingredients, the greater the probability of success. Also, since these ingredients come in subjective degrees rather than in scientific measurable quantities, you must be a good artist who can adapt flexibly to your client.

The next chapter section explains why the hypnotherapist needs more than basic skills plus a script book. (If you do not plan on using hypnosis for therapeutic purposes, you might wish to skip to the next chapter.)

Are the Ingredients Enough?

This book provides a basic understanding of trance management techniques; but when the subconscious resists positive suggestions, the hypnotherapist needs to have both width and depth of training ... both in the basic techniques of hypnosis as well as with hypnotherapy techniques. The reason is because of the "blocks" mentioned at the top of this page (also called *old tapes*, though not all old tapes are negative). The subconscious often *blocks* the ability to believe in goal achievement. If these blocks are left undiscovered, results from hypnotic suggestion alone may be only temporary at best.

Unfortunately, helping clients achieve goals is not as simple as successfully guiding them into hypnosis with the hypnotic formula and giving post-hypnotic suggestions. If it were, this book would be the complete updated version of the Charles Tebbetts Hypnotism Training Course; and the skilled hypnotist could help most of the people most of the time simply by having a good script book.

There is much more for the professional to know and use beyond simply learning a few hypnotic techniques ... but even the successful therapist using hypnosis must still build a good foundation by learning the basics first. Even the experienced therapist could lose the opportunity to help a client if that client pops up out of the hypnotic state, unless that therapist is skilled in trance management techniques. Unfortunately, many hypnotherapy training programs are weak in teaching basic techniques. This book helps fill that gap.

The advanced text, *The Art of Hypnotherapy*, is devoted to the various client-centered rapid change techniques that Charles Tebbetts used so successfully throughout his career – techniques which help to discover subconscious blocks and release them. That book contains some of my own techniques as well as others that have been used for decades. Before moving on, however, I advise my students to MASTER basic techniques with *confidence* and *competence*.

My teacher had us all jump right into the water at this point by going into suggestibility tests and an induction; but first, let's explore some of the history of hypnosis. With the hypnotic formula now in mind, we may well wonder just how the history of this art might be entirely different had our pioneers understood the vital roles of *belief, imagination, conviction, and expectation* rather than simply studying and researching hypnotism as a science.

Chapter 3

Hypnosis: Yesterday and Today

How has the history of hypnosis influenced its present? Does the history of hypnotism validate it as a science, or as an art, or both? Should we analytically research the history of hypnosis simply to examine its scientific aspects, or would it be wiser to consider how the history of hypnosis might be different if it had been done as an art? And will hypnotism survive as an art, or as a science, or as both?

Music could most certainly be examined and analyzed into a pure science of mathematics. One could create countless presentations on the components of the musical scale, harmonics, musical timing, etc., etc., etc.; and there are excellent teachers of all aspects of music, including its history. But when it gets down to performance time, it is the *artist* performing with "feelings" who reaches in and touches our emotions. Music that is mathematically correct can still leave the listener cold when no *artistic feeling* exists, even with all the notes performed accurately and in proper timing!

The Purpose of this Chapter

Since this book is written primarily to be a "how to" presentation about the *art* of hypnosis rather than as a scientific study, some people might wonder why a chapter on the history of hypnosis is even included.

First, I believe it's important for the professional hypnotherapist to be able to discuss some aspects of hypnosis history intelligently, for in so doing we can quite often "win over" a client who might otherwise be skeptical or resistant. We do not have to become experts at the history of an art, be it hypnosis or music, in order to master the performance of that art; but it's also unwise for any hypnotist to be uninformed of the amazing history of hypnosis.

Even though the use of hypnosis was common with many primitive civilizations (though not by the name *hypnosis*), its true nature still seems like a mystery to most people even to this day – as is evidenced by the movies.

The long and often unhappy history of hypnotism demonstrates how *belief, imagination, expectation and conviction* are woven in throughout time – and how ignorance of these vital ingredients of hypnosis resulted in incorrect theories. By glancing at the origin and historical background of some of those early theories of various trance forms, the resulting confusion becomes evident – often providing some interesting conversation with some of your clients as well as with other interested hypnotherapists. The "up side" of all this, however, is that some wonderful benefits have taken place throughout time for many fortunate people on the receiving end of hypnotic research – and enough advances have been made to keep the interest alive.

Hypnotism still has its scientific aspects. It has its experimenters and pioneers, its lucky guessers, and its martyrs – and they have all left their marks on the history of hypnosis.

The information that follows in this chapter comes partly from my own studies and research, partly from personal knowledge of certain individuals, and partly from material I received from some unpublished typed notes from research done by Charles Tebbetts and others.

Possible Origins of Hypnosis

How old is hypnosis? Many might find this hard to believe, but as early as 3,000 B.C., the Egyptians had knowledge of and were using hypnotism, as is proven by hieroglyphics found on tombs of that period. The Greeks also understood it, as well as the Mayas of South America. It was also used by Hindu fakirs, the Chinese teachers of religion, the Persian magi, the Celtic druids and African witch doctors. Perhaps it goes back to prehistoric times, handed down by various rituals.

Some people believe that hypnosis was spontaneously discovered in each civilization of the world as its history unfolded, and that it will become known in any group of people, in any setting. Why, then, is it still a mystery today? Hollywood is not totally to blame.

First, humans are primarily greedy by nature, and pioneers were not exceptions. In all likelihood the first hypnotists soon became the first witch doctors, wise men, shamans, and so on (or vice versa), and the knowledge of the art was jealously guarded – shrouding it in mysticism and religion.

Another reason the lack of knowledge of hypnotism is even more inherent in humans is due to our inborn trait to fear, ridicule, or turn our noses up at that which we don't understand; but every science in the world has had to travel the same hard road from disbelief through fear, to common acceptance. For example, consider how people laughed at the Wright brothers. Most people then thought that if God intended man to fly, he would have given man wings! Now we accept airplanes as a part of life. Even electricity was considered "demonic" power in the not too distant past.

Is it surprising, then, that hypnotism, still considered an occult science by many, should take so long to gain recognition and wide scale acceptance? Since the dawn of history, its secrets have been kept from the average person.

The Hypnotic Pioneers of Yesteryear

Today hypnosis is emerging both as a science and an art; however, the fact that it has slowly become considered a science by the scientific community is because increasing numbers of its proponents have become more scientific in their approaches.

There are literally thousands of people who have contributed to the advancement of hypnotism. Those who are recognized by the scientific community are the ones who took a more scientific approach. However, there are others whose contributions also deserve places in history. Some historical researchers categorize the hypnotic pioneers into four groups, discussed as follows ...

1. The Early Unscientific Group
    This group includes most of those who experimented with hypnosis without knowing it under that name. They share in common the fact that they generally misunderstood the things that they were accomplishing; and instead laid their achievements to magic, or magnetism, divine power, etc.

    They include Genghis Kahn, who used *group suggestion* to create hallucinations. Also included are: Albertus Magnum, Roger Bacon, Raymond Lully, Pico della Mirandola, Paracelsus, Holinotius, Robert Fludd, Father Kirchner, Maxwell, Burcq, and Father Hell, as well as names of people who never found their way into the history books. They also include the seers and sages of Greece, who seem to have been the ancient leaders in self-hypnosis, as well as the ancient Egyptians, and probably tribal "witch doctors" dating back to prehistoric times. And there are some hypnotherapists, including myself, who believe that Jesus used hypnosis with many whom He healed.

2. The Semi-Scientific Group
    This group started experimenting and researching hypnotism as a science, although some of the people in this group never heard the term "hypnosis" during their lifetimes.

    A famous pioneer of trance was Anton Mesmer, whom most people call the "Father of Hypnosis." Others include Father Gassner, the Marquis De Puysegur, as well as James Martin Charcot, a famous man to even modern hypnotists, but who was still years behind his own time in the study of hypnosis; yet some believe that he belongs in this group despite his identification of the depth levels of hypnosis.

These famous hypnotic pioneers and their work will be discussed later in this chapter.

3. The Scientific Group
    The scientific group, also discussed later in this chapter, includes those who first removed hypnosis from the realms of "mysticism" and started experimenting with what hypnosis could actually do. Elliotson, Braid and Esdaile made much progress toward establishing its use in medicine – ending the first dark age of hypnosis. And while they did make a few mistakes, they were still many years ahead of their time; so they deserve their places in fame as scientific investigators of hypnosis.

    Other scientific pioneers include Liebault, Bernheim, Brewer and Freud – even though Freud was responsible for another dark age of hypnosis.

4. The Modern Groups
    The modern groups should include both those who teach and promote hypnotherapy as an art and/or a profession of its own as well as those who research it as a science. But there seems to be a division or gulf today between the scientific community and those many thousands of dedicated full-time hypnotherapists who are and have been successful with helping clients change their lives. So you could say that we have the *modern scientific* group and the *modern artistic* group.

    Among the 20th century scientific researchers, one name shines brilliantly above all others – *Milton Erickson, M.D.*

    There are many other 20th century hypnotic researchers and experimenters. Their names are too numerous to mention here, although some are mentioned later in this chapter.

    Also, we must consider the modern artistic group (what some in the scientific community call "lay hypnotism"). This legitimate hypnotherapy profession of men and women dedicated to helping people almost exclusively with hypnotherapy has produced its own superstars. Names like Ormond McGill and Charles Tebbetts are now already legends, as well as Rexford North. These men were considered *masters of the art*. Some masters of hypnosis in the artistic group have formed professional hypnotherapy associations and/or dedicated themselves to helping people through the art of hypnosis. They will also be discussed later in this chapter.

There is some overlap between the two modern groups, as some of the 20th century researchers of hypnosis did not obtain the usual advanced degrees so common to today's scientific researchers and many earlier pioneers.

Likewise, some fine people with outstanding credentials have also recognized hypnosis as an art and have accepted the validity of hypnotherapists who are *competent artists* even though they might lack the advanced academic degrees. Several of them have even gotten directly involved with some of the professional hypnotherapy associations.

Now let's look more closely at some of these pioneers of both the science and art of hypnotism – and their contributions to hypnosis. The pages that follow are only intended to provide an overview of how the lives and work of these hypnotic pioneers have influenced the history of hypnosis, as well as to show how a simple understanding of the *hypnotic formula* could have greatly influenced the historical course of hypnosis – both yesterday and today.

As you read these pages, be sure to look for our friends: *imagination, belief, expectation and conviction.*

Hypnotic Pioneers of the 18th Century

We will start our discussion of 18th century hypnotic pioneers with a famous name from the semi-scientific group: Anton Mesmer.

Franz Anton Mesmer

Mesmer is probably the most famous name in the entire history of hypnosis, even though he never heard of the art or the science by that name.

As the first man ever to try to explain scientifically what he was doing, he is often given credit for being the "Father of Hypnosis," a title he shares with two other men. Even today we speak of "mesmerizing" someone, and the hypnotherapy community still bears many references to him and his work, as an undeniable tribute.

Mesmer was born in Iznang, Germany, on May 23, 1734, on the Bordensee, or Lake of Constance. Because this lake is also bordered by Switzerland and Austria, some publications list him as being born in either of these countries, or on other dates, due to the inaccuracy of records kept at that time.

He first studied medicine in Vienna, where he became a practicing physician.

After seeing a demonstration of magnetic cures by Father Maximilian Hell in 1774, he began his experiments with magnets. He apparently borrowed his first magnets from Father Hell. Then, in 1766, Mesmer wrote his doctoral dissertation, *"De Planetarum Influxu"* (The Planetorium Flux) in which he first formulated his theory concerning the influence of planets upon the human body. He believed that a general sort of magnetic fluid pervaded nature and the human body, and that this fluid must be evenly distributed throughout the body for wellness. He postulated that our own bodies were like magnets with poles at either end – and that bringing a magnet close to the body would help balance and harmonize this magnetic fluid around us. His theory was first called "animal gravitation" and eventually became known as "animal magnetism." Although his theories intrigued many, he also blended astrology and metaphysics into his theories – which widened the credibility gap with the skeptics.

His first subject was Franzl Oesterlin, a young girl who was a friend of Mesmer's wife. The girl was a victim of hysteria and combined convulsions, with symptoms of vomiting, temporary blindness, attacks of paralysis, hallucinations, inability to pass urine, violent toothache and "other terrible symptoms," to quote Mesmer. Magnets were tied to her feet and hung around her neck and "*a hot piercing pain rose along her legs from her feet and ended with an intenser spasm in the upper rim of the iliac bone. Here this pain was united with an equally agonizing one which flowed from both sides of the breast, shot pains up to the head and united in the roots of the hair. The patient felt a burning sensation in all her joints. At certain parts of her body the magnetic stream seemed to be interrupted, even to become more intense. She was soon insensitive to all the magnets and cured of her attacks.*"

The cure was permanent.

Now let's consider what happened ... Magnets at that time were new and mysterious, and some *believed* that they had great powers. The subject respected them and was *convinced* that they would produce results. And because results were *expected*, results were produced!

Also, at that time, pain was considered necessary for healing. What the magnets did, then, through our friends *belief, conviction and expectation*, was to produce a quick, intense pain that did the job of beating psychological symptoms.

Before long, Mesmer discovered that magnets were not essential to the "cure" and instead came to believe that the results were due to an invisible, voluminous fluid which permeated everything and was affected by the position of the planets.

He soon modified his magnetism theories to include the fact that he somehow became endowed with much more "magnetic fluid" than other people – though everyone did have a certain amount.

Mesmer's fame grew quickly, and he magnetized many; and, as is easy to believe, the other practicing physicians became furious and labeled him a *quack!*

But he just kept right on with his work.

Unfortunately for the evolution of hypnotism, Mesmer *did not know* that his "cures" were entirely due to his artistry of inducing a guided self-trance, helping patients actually use the power of their own subconscious minds for their cures – so his first defeat left him without a good response.

In attempting to cure a neurotic blind girl, Maria Theresa Paradies, pianist and protégé of the empress, he managed to help her restore her sight but found himself unable to explain her loss of equilibrium – which angered her parents greatly. Her father came to Mesmer's clinic demanding he release her immediately. She begged to stay; but her father drew his blade with his demand, and she went into convulsions and lost her sight again, never to regain it, although there was nothing physically wrong with her eyes.

Mesmer's critics naturally took advantage of this incident; and a commission was appointed to investigate. They did so – for three years – and then decided that Mesmer was a danger to Vienna and gave him only two days to leave town.

He then moved to Paris, where he invited leading scientists to witness his demonstrations, and encouraged the poorer classes to come to his clinic for treatment. The slow, discouraging responses resulted in his moving on to Belgium in 1781.

Mozart became a Mesmer fan, and after Mozart's insistence, Mesmer returned to Paris and bought a hotel on the Rue Mootmarte, where he turned away from the science of magnetizing people, and became a showman practicing his cures as an *art* – causing no small stir in France.

His clinic itself became a showplace in Paris – where getting mesmerized became as popular as going up in hot air balloons. Mesmer developed the legendary *bacquet*, a monstrosity which would even be the envy of some modern showmen today! It was a round contraption, roughly a foot high, with a seating capacity of about 30. There were holes in the top where subjects could grasp iron rods and receive the "magnetic flow" and go with the flow. Inside were numerous bottles which he had previously filled with the all-important, invisible, healing "magnetic fluid" – which, of course, flowed from one of his finger tips. The entire scenario was enhanced with music, unusual lightings, and the presence of highly suggestible subjects, so that even a skeptic generally found it easy to trance out into convulsions by grasping one of the iron rods. At times, Mesmer "magnetized" empty envelopes which, when opened, would produce a convulsion. Couldn't Hollywood make this an interesting scene in a movie?

All this show business again brought him under public scorn in France – so much so that cartoons were published during his life depicting Mesmer with the face and ears of a donkey while magnetizing a woman, with the caption: "LE DOIGT MAGIQUE OU LE MAGNÉTISME ANIMAL." Some cartoons were so demeaning that they depicted both Mesmer and his followers as dogs!

Mesmer remained in Paris this time until a commission appointed by King Louis XVI and headed by Benjamin Franklin investigated his work and turned in an unfavorable report. One of the experiments Franklin observed was with a woman who drank a mesmerized cup of water which *she believed to be normal.* Nothing happened. Yet when she drank a normal cup that *she believed* had been *mesmerized,* she tranced out!

Another experiment involved trees which had been mesmerized. Again, the subject failed to trance out at the correct tree – but instead went into convulsions when touching the tree that he *believed* had been magnetized. Franklin stated that Mesmer was a fraud, as all his cures and theatrical results were caused by *imagination.* Any of us could have come to the same conclusion.

I wonder if Franklin had any idea that a day would come when an entire profession of hypnotherapy would rely so heavily on his correct observation! What is seldom disclosed is that Franklin believed that more experiments were appropriate to discover the impact of imagination; but he was shipped back to America once Mesmer's peers got what they wanted.

At any rate, Mesmer unfortunately did not understand the role of imagination in his successes, and was forced into retirement in

Switzerland, where he lived quietly and sadly, occasionally treating his neighbors until his death in 1815. Far before his death, he lost control of mesmerism, as spiritualists blended it with spiritualism.

Had either Mesmer or any other early key pioneers of hypnosis really understood the vital role of even some of the ingredients of the hypnotic formula, *belief, imagination, expectation and conviction,* the entire history of hypnosis would have changed course! It seems tragic that even the 19th century pioneers failed to learn from Mesmer's mistake. Why couldn't they make the same correct observation made by Benjamin Franklin in the late 18th century?

One of Mesmer's direct descendants was interviewed in the early 1990s by Penny Dutton Raffa, founder of the International Hypnosis Hall of Fame. It is my hope that the contents of this interview will become available in written form sometime in the future. Unfortunately, due to the founder's health problems, the International Hypnosis Hall of Fame went into hibernation after the dawn of the 21st century. Only time will tell whether this organization gets revived. In my professional opinion, what Mrs. Raffa founded must survive.

Father Gassner

Father Gassner, a Catholic priest, was contemporary with Mesmer (1727–1779), and was also active in hypnosis. He apparently worked briefly with Mesmer, according to at least one historian. Father Gassner mastered the art of suggestion as a means of faith healing, and was perhaps the first of the modern faith healers.

On at least one occasion, Gassner lowered a woman's pulse rate and breathing until two horrified doctors (who were invited to the demonstration) pronounced her dead. Then, two and a half minutes later, he returned her bodily functions to normal, and "brought her back to life" again.

His parish couldn't help but have a *belief* that God had endowed him with heavenly powers, and the psychological advantage he then had was their tremendous *conviction* that something would happen!

As a religious authority as well, Gassner worked under the most favorable conditions possible for hypnotic response. People *believed* that he represented God's authority over them, and therefore *expected* things to happen when Father Gassner spoke. (Does this sound familiar?)

Imagine this scenario and its dramatics: He did his trance induction in a dimly lit cathedral, circling his subjects while carrying a candle-lit, diamond-studded crucifix, and muttering "sleep" suggestions in Latin. And because of their *belief*, his subjects could easily *imagine* the power of God working through the priest! Thus, even difficult subjects were sent instantly to sleep by the touch of the cross, while the mere presence of this cross was enough to hypnotize most subjects.

Gassner's average trance induction time was an almost unbelievable seven seconds, again proving the effectiveness of *belief, imagination, expectation and conviction.*

Gassner was one of the first men to produce a quiet sleep in the hypnotic state, rather than the usual trance convulsion. Because of this great difference between his methods and those of the "magnetizers," however, he was not considered to be a scientific researcher. Perhaps he most closely parallels the modern artistic group.

Marquis Chastenet de Puysegur

A former student of Mesmer's, and one of Mesmer's most unscientific followers, Marquis Chastenet de Puysegur (also spelled *Pursegur*) lived and experimented in Buzancy, France. He evolved Mesmer's theories about magnetism into what became known as directed magnetism.

Puysegur formulated the theory that the prime factor producing magnetism was the magnetizer himself. So another common mistake remained – the assumption that the power resided with the hypnotist rather than in the mind of the subject.

Because of the above mistaken opinion, the Marquis decided that the magnets were not necessary – so he would "magnetize" an elm tree and get results with people visiting that elm tree.

Imagine that! The local populace could go enjoy the latest in trance convulsions even in the Marquis's absence (while he apparently did more important things).

Would you agree that the **hypnotic formula** was at work here in the minds of people "magnetized" by a tree? If one *believed* that a certain tree had been magnetized, and he/she could easily *imagine* becoming magnetized by that same tree, and therefore *expected* to be magnetized, wouldn't hypnosis occur even if it was the wrong tree? Franklin had already observed someone trancing out after touching the wrong tree during his experiments with Mesmer's work.

Hollywood could really create an interesting scenario showing the Marquis making his magnetic passes around those he magnetized, and could then add more dramatics by including an ominous looking elm tree. Add in some mysterious music and a few dark clouds, etc., and I'm certain the effects would be quite dramatic on screen. (Sometimes my motion picture family heritage influences my methods of telling stories!)

A far more important contribution from Puysegur came when he discovered the sleep-like trance state and gave it the name "somnambulism" which remains to this day. This first happened in 1784 when a young shepherd, Victor Race, fell into a quiet sleep instead of the usual convulsion while tied to one of the "magnetized" trees. Puysegur found that the young boy could respond to suggestions while still appearing to be asleep.

According to Robert Darnton, author of *Mesmerism and the End of the Enlightenment in France*, the Marquis became very famous, even gaining support from some in government.

> *By the autumn of 1784, the Marquis de Puysegur was mesmerizing on a huge scale with the enthusiastic support of local officials in Bayonne, and accounts of his feats circulated throughout the nation along with records of cures performed by straight mesmerizing. (p. 58)*

After this, however, Puysegur went on to experiment with E.S.P. and other theories unacceptable to the scientific community. However, he still goes down in history for the discovery of the somnambulistic trance, as well as for being the first man in medical history to experiment with diagnosis of illness during trance – although his diagnoses were through the medium of the sixth sense and frequently incorrect.

But was Puysegur's decision to experiment with E.S.P. his biggest mistake?

In *Hypnosis: The Cognitive-Behavioral Perspective* (p. 79), Nicholas Spanos and John Chaves state the following:

> *Mesmer and Puysegur claimed that hypnotic phenomena depended upon the special prowess or supernatural skills of the hypnotist, under whose agency the "magnetized" person behaved as a virtual automaton.*

As mentioned earlier, the Marquis mistakenly believed that his subjects were "under his power" – and somehow there are people even today who still believe that! Again we might ask: how different might the history of hypnosis have been if Mesmer and Puysegur understood that all mesmerism was really *guided self-mesmerism?*

Perhaps the problem with that perception is that it takes much of the science out of the process, and requires much more artistry – especially with resistant subjects. Even today, people still debate the question of who has the power.

Other practitioners of that time

All the way into the first part of the 19th century, many men studied and practiced different types of hypnosis with many different approaches, even though the word "hypnosis" had not yet been coined. Commissions were appointed to investigate their findings and works, with reports that were just as unfavorable as Mesmer's review.

Most of the pioneers of that time followed in Puysegur's shoes, experimenting with clairvoyance and E.S.P., which fueled the fires of the skeptics. Apparently most people with scientific minds want scientific facts and scientific theories – not alternative ideas – even if said alternative ideas provide some benefit to some people. Isn't it interesting, however, that so many of these scientists did explore the areas of E.S.P.? We do not explore these areas in my class, as Charles Tebbetts wanted his course taught in a secular and believable way.

Hypnosis in the 19th Century

Abbe Jose Castodi de Faria

Abbe Faria was one of the first *scientific* experimenters in hypnosis, operating in Paris around 1815. It was he who first formulated many of the theories which were later rediscovered by and credited to other men.

He was the first man we know to have discovered that psychological attitudes had anything to do with a hypnotic condition, and taught that a trance could not be induced against one's will. He also developed the *"fixed-gaze method"* of induction, leading to myriads of induction techniques used then as well as today which are based on eye fixation.

Besides being an investigator into the "whys" of hypnosis, Faria was quite a showman as well; and at that time hypnosis really needed a good "public relations" man. He was doing very well in both his jobs of discovering hypnotism and selling it to the public, when the incident came that ended his career and cheated him out of virtually all the credit that he so rightly deserves.

Several jealous doctors hired some people to pose as subjects for Faria at a public demonstration, pretending to go into trance very quickly and easily. At the correct psychological moment, they jumped up and announced that they were only shamming, and falsely claimed that Faria had hired them. Naturally this disgusting product of jealousy discredited Faria, and he lost all of the recognition he justly deserved.

John Elliotson

John Elliotson, born in 1791, was a professor of theory and practice at University Hospital in London, England. He became interested in magnetism through a Richard Chenevix, a student of Faria's, and learned it from Baron de Potet.

Because of the nature and methods of his research, this pioneer definitely deserves to be considered a pioneer among the scientific group.

Beginning his experiments in 1837, Elliotson found that his patients could undergo major surgery without agony, and he applied these techniques whenever possible. This incurred the wrath of his fellow physicians, who clung to a firm belief that pain was necessary for healing. Consequently, this made many doctors eager to discredit Elliotson. Because he also believed in clairvoyance, they used this as extra ammunition and put his real work into the same category.

Despite open criticism and disguised enmity, Elliotson continued using and promoting "magnetism," and many younger doctors displayed great interest in his work. He gained so many followers that he was forced to perform many of his operations in the hospital amphitheater to seat all those who wished to attend.

In addition to using hypnosis in major operations, Elliotson also used "prestige suggestion" for some direct cures. He also conducted some experiments with trance diagnosis and predictions; yet he still probably did more actually to promote hypnotism to the medical world in a scientific way than any of his forerunners.

The medical community continued the attacks on him, however. This soon made him very unpopular with the public – and even less popular with the hospital authorities, who asked him to discontinue his experiments.

Firmly convinced he was right, he refused to stop. After a stormy scene, he left the hospital and university, never to return. Unfortunately, as we might expect, all traces of mesmerism were "cleaned away" behind him – by a specially appointed commission.

Another tragic blow had been aimed at the heart of hypnotism by the scientific community of the time, right at its leading scientific practitioner.

Elliotson continued to fight for medical acceptance of his experiments for over 30 years in any way he could. He published a journal called "Zoist," which indirectly resulted in benefits for thousands of people in later years through the work of James Esdaile. But with most of his work ignored, he died a bitter man in 1868. It's a shame that he couldn't have enjoyed more of the respect he so justly deserved while he was still living. Another great man died without honor.

James Braid

James Braid (1795–1860), a prominent Scottish surgeon, is most famous for coining the word "hypnosis" (derived from the Greek word *hypnos*, meaning sleep).

His work helped advance hypnosis greatly, as he was the first man to be recognized for scientific experimentation into the "whys" of mesmerism. He also developed another eye-fixation type induction technique with the use of bright light, and discovered how to enhance the trance with much more emphasis on vocal suggestions. He believed that the trance depended on the suggestibility of the subject, which could be influenced greatly by vocal suggestions from the hypnotist. This came to be called the *suggestions method*.

For these things Braid is also referred to as the "Father of Hypnosis" – a historic honor also shared with both Mesmer and Liebault.

Braid's hypnotic career began after seeing a "magnetism" demonstration in November of 1841 – and he challenged the mystic claims of Mesmer. He branded the show as an insult to scientific intelligence; but somehow felt compelled to see a demonstration at least one more time before dismissing it as fraud.

Fortunately, the second demonstration convinced him that the magnetizer had the subject under complete control, and Braid's curiosity now motivated him to find out how this was done. The downside, however, was that Braid assumed that the subject was *under the magnetizer's power* – so in spite of his successes, he still followed down one of the same erroneous paths as the earlier pioneers of hypnosis.

After originally dismissing Mesmer's theories as a stubborn collection of old wives' tales, Braid still found himself confronted with a phenomenon without an acceptable explanation of its cause! But he concluded that there must be a physical cause, so he began his research. He theorized that a continued straining of the eyes could, through fatigue, result in a paralysis of the optic nerve centers, causing a condition that would much resemble sleep – thus his great interest in "fixed-gaze" (or eye-fixation) methods.

He experimented by having a friend stare continually at a wine bottle, and in less than three minutes had legitimate proof that magnetism had nothing to do with a mesmeristic sleep. His friend, and later his wife, both proved to be excellent subjects, and Braid's experiments proved to be the indisputable origin of some of the scientific contributions to hypnotism. However, he mistakenly assumed that something physiological took place as a result of the fixed-gaze techniques which created an absence of volition; thus Braid failed to realize that all hypnosis is self-hypnosis.

Also, as happens so often with hypnosis, his conservative British colleagues in the medical community gave him virtually no honor for his work, even though there were many accomplishments. He submitted reports to the British association and offered to do experiments for a special commission, but the offer was formally refused.

While Braid found little or no honor in his home country, his articles stirred considerable interest in France. Yet Azam, his French disciple who was considered a "quack" in France was lauded highly in England! And the "best minds" of the day did this to these pioneers of hypnosis?

The most important thing to remember about Braid's real contributions to hypnosis is that he was the first to stipulate that hypnotic sleep could be induced by physical agents – also adding that psychological conditions, *belief* and *expectation*, were necessary for successful induction.

It was in 1842 that Braid gave us the word "hypnotism" – which he tried to change later to "monoideism," as he found that the condition could also exist in a state that does not include sleep. However, the first name caught on so well that it remains to this day in spite of many efforts to change it. Even many modern day practitioners attempt to disguise the practice of hypnotism with other names such as "group meditation," "programmed imagery," "guided relaxation," "guided imagery" or "creative visualization," etc.; but the word "hypnosis" is obviously here to stay.

In 1843 Braid published the first work on hypnotism to be known by that name, disclaiming the term "Braidism." And then, in 1847, he discovered "waking hypnosis," accomplishing more in just six years than had been done in over a century by hundreds of other experimenters.

Finally, in 1848, Braid wandered into phrenology and hypnogenic zones, ending research that would be considered valid by the scientific community. So yet another scientist exploring hypnosis in a scientific way explored unknown realms. This leaves some people curious ...

James Esdaile

While Braid was making quantum leaps with hypnosis, another Scottish doctor, James Esdaile (1808–1859), was experimenting and gaining permanent recognition in the history of hypnosis. Stationed in Hoogly, India, Esdaile used hypnosis in surgery with astounding results; and even today many would say that his work with applied hypnosis almost borders on the fantastic.

Esdaile submitted reports at the end of 1846 indicating that he had performed several thousand minor operations and about 300 major ones, including 19 amputations, all painlessly. Due mostly to the removal of post-operative shock through hypnosis, he cut the 50 percent mortality rate of that time down to less than 8 percent! (One book even reported less than 5 percent.) The Medical Association actually accepted his report, and he was assigned to the Calcutta hospital to continue "mesmeristic" operations.

While the Association considered mesmerism taboo at University Hospital, mesmerism could quite easily be expected to work for the uneducated masses in India. They were right, of course. In India, long known as the home of occult sciences, Esdaile was assured of success from the very beginning because of the common *belief* system. Later, when Esdaile returned home, he was unable to duplicate his work because of lack of belief and negative expectation; so his career went down the same dark path of discouragement taken by Elliotson.

Dave Elman gave Esdaile respect by referring to an ultra-deep hypnotic state as the Esdaile state (Chapter 13 of his book, *Hypnotherapy*, is entitled: "The Esdaile State").

Dr. Burcq

A French physician, Dr. Burcq, played a minor but interesting part in the development of hypnotism about this time, although his name is rarely connected with hypnosis.

Dr. Burcq developed the science of "metaloscopy," which received recognition and respectability in medical ranks long before hypnotism did.

In metaloscopy, the sick were treated by the application of various metals, externally, to the afflicted portions of the anatomy. Iron was used for drawing out postural lesions; lead placed over the heart was the specific metal used in anemia, and so on. When these substances were applied and allowed to remain for various periods of time, spectacular changes were supposed to occur. In physical illness, it must be asked if the same changes would not have been affected through the body's own curative powers; in psychosomatic illnesses, one could easily assume that the cure was brought about by the *expectation* alone; but consider... How much of this success might also be due to the effect of the other components of the hypnotic formula – *belief, imagination, and conviction?*

Even today some alternative therapies use pendulums and various gadgets for diagnosing, but it is not recognized as scientific. When cures take place, it may be due to the placebo effect – which has the same components of the hypnotic formula. Or, said another way, perhaps these people are cured by *their own mind power!* And if this is true, then perhaps Dr. Burcq was indeed a facilitator of the *art* of trance induction, helping many of his patients use the power of their own minds to heal themselves.

The Nancy School of Thought: Bernheim and Liebault

In 1864 a country doctor, Ambroise August Liebault, settled in Nancy, France. He established his practice there, treating patients either hypnotically or with medicine.

Because his hypnotic treatments were free, they naturally became popular.

These treatments were only about ten minutes long, and Dr. Liebault made it quite clear that he had no supernatural power. He is the first man we know of to have taught that hypnosis is purely a matter of suggestion – so he courageously stepped foot on a new path!

Hippolyte Bernheim, a professor of medicine at the Nancy Medical School, wrote an article discrediting Liebault as a fraud; but a visit to Liebault's clinic convinced him otherwise, because the doctor's methods were gaining results. He then introduced Liebault's methods at his own clinic with equal or greater success.

Soon he returned to Nancy, joined Liebault, and with him founded history's most renowned center for hypnotic healing. He claimed success in 85 percent of his cases, claiming success even in a lead poisoning case.

On original cases, Bernheim kept very careful records, and published many of them *"De la Suggestion"* in 1884. In 1886 he published *"Suggestive Therapeutics,"* – which became widely used as a guide to medical hypnosis.

Bernheim and Liebault are usually referred to as the founders of the School of Nancy, a school both in actuality and in thought. The theory of this school is that even the eye fatigue of Braid is unnecessary, and that hypnosis is a purely subjective thing. In other words, they correctly determined that psychological forces rather than physical forces caused hypnosis. As this theory is now generally accepted, we can say that the art of hypnosis took another giant leap forward.

Perhaps their biggest mistake, however, was in still believing that once a person was hypnotized, the power was with the physician rather than the person in hypnosis. On page 100 of *The Young Freud* (Billa Zanuso), the author says:

The basic theory of the Nancy school was that everything which occurred under hypnosis was caused by the physician's power of suggestion over the patient.

If Bernheim and Liebault had realized that all hypnosis is really guided self-hypnosis, and that the power was really within the mind of the person being hypnotized, how would this have altered the course of hypnotism? The hypnotic formula must take place *within the mind of the person entering hypnosis*, not within the mind of the hypnotist – as was evidenced by Esdaile's lack of success in duplicating hypnotic anesthesia in Great Britain as he had done in India.

The School of Salpetriere: Charcot

At the same time Bernheim and Liebault were studying hypnotism in Nancy, Dr. James Martin Charcot experimented with it in his clinic at Salpetriere. He was the first one to identify and label the various levels of hypnotic depth.

Although one of the most advanced neurologists of his day, Charcot made several mistakes when he approached the new subject. Basically, he believed that hypnosis was a phenomena that could best be studied with patients of hysteria – and taught that hypnosis itself was a pathological state. In short, his view was that physical action was the cause of hypnosis rather than psychological suggestion, so his theories were in conflict with those of Liebault and Bernheim. Two other beliefs he had were in the somatic induction of hypnotic sleep by the touching of "hypnogenic zones," and in the validity of Dr. Burcq's metaloscopy theory.

Even though Charcot's basic ideas about hypnosis may have been incorrect, he made an important discovery in recognizing and naming various depth levels of hypnosis.

In 1878, Charcot and his pupils at the academy proved these stages of hypnotic sleep by showing that the hypnotized subject is capable of showing different symptoms and passing different "tests" in each stage. This was the first attempt at a scientific classification of trance phenomena, and it is fortunate for the later history of hypnosis that Charcot adapted it. (It is reflected in modern times in the famous Davis-Husband scale of hypnotic depths, the frequently used LeCron-Bordeaux scale, and so on.)

It was in Charcot's treatise, "On the Distinct Nororaphy of the Different Phases of Sciences Comprised Under the Name of Hypnotism," that the three widely-accepted depths of hypnosis were first named and defined.

The names that Charcot applied to the stages, in order, are *LETHARGY, CATALEPSY*, and *SOMNAMBULISM*. Various hypnotists use other scales composing four, five, seven, or more stages of trance depth, but the three-step scale devised by Charcot continues to be the most practical today.

Charcot became recognized throughout the medical world for his contributions to the field of neurology, and his acceptance of hypnotism caused many doctors of that time to likewise accept it. His misconceptions were also unfortunately accepted, causing some time lapse in discovering more of the truths about hypnosis; still, another huge step forward had been taken.

19th Century Hypnosis at Its Height

Liebault, Bernheim, and Charcot inspired many new men to enter the study of hypnotism at this time, and both public and medical acceptance of hypnotism as a science throughout Europe became a reality. Even though modern methods of hypnotherapy were not thought of yet, great strides were made in almost every medical field through the application of hypnosis by these scientific pioneers who explored various medical uses of hypnotism. The names of others who did important research or made interesting reports are too numerous to mention here.

Again, let's balance our enthusiasm with caution, as most of these earlier successes were due to the mistaken *belief* that the patient experiencing hypnosis was subject to the suggestion of the opera-tor. Since this was the *expectation* on the part of both the subject as well as the hypnotist, we can only speculate on how many successes were really the result of the "placebo" effect – especially since most of these pioneers used *prestige suggestion* alone, a procedure which is allowable considering the much smaller understanding of psychodynamics at that time. Also, because most patients were *convinced* that the physician was an authority on the use of hypnotism, they could easily *imagine* being under the power of the medical authority of the day. (What others refer to as *prestige suggestion* – the use of suggestion alone to bring about changes in a person's life – was called "Band-Aid therapy" by Charles Tebbetts.)

As mentioned above, if a person in hypnosis could *imagine* direct suggestion alone "curing" him/her, and the *belief* brought about a total *conviction* that hypnotic suggestion would make a change, and the *expectation* was for the cure to be lasting, then the changes would be permanent. In practicing hypnotism for over six decades, Charles Tebbetts came to the conclusion that direct suggestion alone will not permanently remove a symptom unless one has a strong motivating desire to change *and* the problem is *not* the result of an emotionally traumatic event. In light of this, he felt that one should use hypnosis to help a client discover and release the *cause* of a problem.

Even though they mistakenly thought the subject was "under their power," had these men of the early and mid-1800s used hypnosis to look for *causes* of problems (as done by *competently trained* hypnotherapists today), and then build upon belief, imagination, conviction and expectation – rather than simply suggesting symptom removal – hypnotherapy would have most certainly taken a different course in the 20th century. Instead, even with their breakthroughs, their lack of understanding of important key elements of the art of hypnosis resulted in hypnosis arriving at a historical crossroad – and Freud took the wrong fork in the road.

Breuer and Freud: Hypnosis advancement and regression

In 1880, a Dr. Joseph Breuer was treating a hysterical girl when he found that the patient could speak distinctly and rationally in the hypnotic state, but had far greater resistance to personal conversation in the conscious state. He attempted direct questioning as to the *cause* of one of her symptoms – an inability to drink water from a cup – and found that she could *remember the cause*. This was impossible for her in the waking state. Her inability to drink stemmed from a time when she was nauseated by watching a dog drinking from a cup she had used; and when this fact was explained to her in the waking state, she both remembered the incident and regained her ability to drink from a cup! In other words, once the basic cause of her psychosomatic symptom was discovered, her symptom vanished.

This is the basis of both hypnoanalysis and psychoanalysis. It was a use of a hypnotherapy technique other than direct prestige suggestion, and produced much more lasting results.

Another contribution Breuer made to the field of hypnoanalysis was the discovery of free *association*. Using this, it is possible for the analyst to get information which cannot otherwise be reached due to resistance, modesty, mental blocks, or insufficient trance depth. It was the ability of free association to be used in light stages of sleep that soon led to the discovery by Sigmund Freud of psychoanalysis.

Freud, attracted to research by Breuer, had already been a student of hypnosis at both the Nancy and Salpetriere schools; but he didn't believe everything he was taught.

According to Billa Zanuso, author of *The Young Freud*, he disagreed with Charcot in two important areas. First, Freud discarded the theory about hypnosis being useful only for hysterics. Second, he did not believe that deep levels of hypnosis were necessary for change; but, rather, suggestions could be accepted and past events recalled even in a light state of hypnosis. Unfortunately for the future of hypnotism at that time, however, Freud was apparently a poor artist at the skill of inductions. He admitted that he wearied quickly of the "monotony of the sleep suggestions." (Note that some experts today believe that deeper levels provide better long-term probabilities of success; but even now this is still debated.)

When working with one patient, Freud was unable to produce a hypnotic trance, and had almost reached the point of despair when – in desperation – he hit on the idea of trying free association in the waking state. The case proved to be successful, and Freud apparently welcomed the opportunity to drop hypnosis from his methods, creating and publicizing the technique of *psychoanalysis*. He then taught that psychoanalysis was now "the executor of the estate left by hypnotism."

Since resistance could be overcome without hypnosis, another "selling point" of hypnotism was lost, and Freud now led a general abandonment of its use. Yet, according to James Russell, Ph.D., author of *Psychosemantic Parenthetics* (and researcher of hypnosis), Freud still used forms of hypnosis even after he supposedly abandoned its use. Yet he now discouraged many practitioners from using hypnosis by teaching that psychosomatic symptoms served an important economic function in the psychic life of the patient, so that the use of hypnosis by prestige suggestions to remove the symptoms was irrational.

As we know today, suggestion alone is often insufficient for permanent results even during deep hypnotic states; thus, the discovery of numerous "relapses" and conversion symptoms during that time almost succeeded in dealing the art of hypnosis a death blow. From literally thousands of articles written about it annually, the number dwindled to several dozen.

Despite its terrific advancement, Freud managed to give hypnosis a hypnotic regression backwards in time – with its flames of interest just barely flickering.

The Most Common Mistake of the Pioneers

There is a common thread running through the accounts discussed so far in this chapter: all these researchers believed that *they* had the power – and that the persons subject to their experiments gave up their free will and *subjected* themselves to the operator (hence the word *subject*).

Nicholas Spanos and John Chaves wrote the following in their book, *Hypnosis: The Cognitive-Behavioral Perspective*:

> *The history of hypnosis contains repeated references to the so-called classic suggestion effect, the apparent absence of volition in the performances of hypnosis subjects. This apparent lack of agency was not problematic to those scientists and practitioners who subscribed to the mental state theory. Given that the person was regarded as an object or organism, the scientific observer would merely record evidence of purported happenings within the organism. It was thus irrelevant to raise the question whether the subject willfully performed a particular action. (p. 403)*

Note carefully that last statement: "It was thus irrelevant to raise the question whether the subject willfully performed a particular action." The authors also point out on page 79 of the same work the fact that both Mesmer and Puysegur claimed that results depended upon the "special prowess or supernatural skills" of the hypnotist, causing the "magnetized" person to behave as a virtual automaton. They go on to say:

> *... an inspection of influential writings from the latter half of the nineteenth century compels the conclusion that helplessness on the part of the subject was seen as an essential feature of successful hypnosis. The idea that a loss of volition constituted ultimate proof that the subject was hypnotized emanated from the influential hypnosis theories of the day. (p. 79)*

Was this client-centered hypnotherapy? I don't think so!

Perhaps if any of our pioneers had understood all the components of the hypnotic formula they might have come to the conclusion that all hypnosis is guided self-hypnosis, or vice versa. Or had even Freud taken a quantum leap forward and realized the above, both the history of hypnosis and the history of psychology would have been forever altered.

Now the 20th century dawned with hypnosis virtually in the dark ages again – but this century would find an amazing hypnotic evolution taking place in its latter decades.

20th Century Hypnosis

Janet, Bramwell, Sidis, and Coué

During the time between Freud's discoveries and World War I, only the efforts of a few interested men kept hypnosis from being forgotten entirely. Even Liebault, who had done so much with it, hardly regarded it as having any real or lasting value. The few who carried the torch include Pierre Janet in France, J. Milne Bramwell in Great Britain, and Boris Sidis in the USA. Émile Coué also made some lasting contributions, especially with his theories of waking hypnosis and autosuggestion, and some call him the father of self-hypnosis.

The light shines again on hypnosis

After the first world war, there were many cases of war neuroses and other trauma caused by the anxiety of war and by a shortage of psychotherapists. The need for qualified doctors was still acute, and an extreme need was evident for a fast method of therapy. In desperation the medical profession turned again to hypnosis, and the answer was there – as it has been since the dawn of time.

Also, as throughout time, entertainers and masters in the art of stage hypnosis – such as Ormond McGill and other stage "magicians" – have preserved public interest in hypnosis through numerous entertaining public demonstrations. Even Charles Tebbetts himself did his share of stage hypnosis during the earlier part of the 20th century.

In the Second World War, hypnosis was again needed in numerous treatments; also, doctors in prisoner-of-war hospitals, denied drugs, were forced to use suggestive anesthesia alone. They were surprised – and pleased – to learn not only that hypnotism worked, but that in most cases the healing was actually promoted. The reports of these men became available after the war; and young doctors, unafraid of new techniques, began applying hypnosis in dentistry, obstetrics, dermatology and other fields. Once again, the use of medical applications of hypnosis was on the upswing.

Dave Elman helped the upswing in the medical community by the middle of this century by teaching hypnosis to many in the medical profession; and the Council on Mental Health of the American Medical Association finally accepted the use of hypnosis in 1958.

Perhaps the most important contributor to the acceptance of both the science and the art of hypnotherapy in the 20th century was a psychiatrist whom some call the *father of counseling hypnotherapy* – who also deserves the title *grandfather of hypnotherapy* – Dr. Milton Erickson.

So great are this man's accomplishments that one could spend years just studying them. People with outstanding professional credentials have examined, analyzed, and written books about the work of Dr. Erickson; and some of his past students have produced an audio cassette of Dr. Erickson's voice – *to go with you!*

What is interesting to note is that high numbers of people with medical backgrounds or other advanced academic degrees approach the work of Dr. Erickson primarily from an analytical standpoint trying to draw analytical conclusions as to why he did certain things the way he did. At the same time, many professional hypnotherapists who approach hypnotherapy more as an art consider Dr. Erickson to be a master of hypnosis who worked *intuitively*.

In the summer of 1991 I was invited to go to Princeton to present a workshop on some of the Tebbetts methods for the International Society of Professional Hypnosis. One of the people attending my workshop was a psychiatrist who told me that he had been a personal friend of Dr. Milton Erickson. When I asked him whether Dr. Erickson worked intuitively as an artist, or purely as a scientist of hypnosis, his answer was: *"Milt was an intuitive master of the art!"* He was both a scientist and an artist.

Besides Milton Erickson, 20th century researchers within the scientific community with advanced degrees who have contributed to hypnosis in a *scientific* manner are people whose names are familiar to most modern hypnotists: Rosen, Abramson, Menninger, Shenek, Magonet, Wolberg, LeCron, Bordeaux, Weitzenhoffer, Erwin (doing amazing things with burn patients), Simonton (contributing outstanding work with cancer patients), and more – who have worked countless hours to research numerous applications of hypnosis.

The American Society of Clinical Hypnosis was eventually born (A.S.C.H.), and hypnosis is now recognized by the American Medical Association as a science that is here to stay. But is hypnosis *only to be done as a science?*

The ART of Hypnotherapy: Birth of a New Profession

As Dr. Erickson began his vitally important work, the seeds were already beginning to grow for the birth of hypnotherapy as an *art* – a profession composed of men and women dedicated to the use of hypnotherapy to help people improve their lives. Although some medical applications of hypnosis are used when done with a written referral (or direct supervision) of an examining physician, there are countless non-medical uses for hypnosis that do not require advanced degrees – such as motivation, habit control, etc.

Countless numbers of clients have been helped by those of us who are trained in the art of hypnosis and call ourselves *hypnotherapists* regardless of academic degrees. Hundreds of thousands of former smokers who no longer smoke strongly demonstrate this fact – as well as countless more whose lives have been improved by non-medical uses of hypnosis. Yet in a strange twist of history repeating itself, some of the worst criticism of professional hypnotherapists comes (even while this book is being revised) from some of the *very same psychological and medical professionals who research and advocate the scientific uses of hypnotism!*

Men and women across the country who devote their lives to the art of hypnotherapy are labeled "lay hypnotists" in a condescending way even though they may have had hundreds of hours of training and many thousands of hours of full-time experience! Yet some 20th century scientific researchers with the advanced degrees have engaged in experiments that are quite insensitive to their subjects – incorporating some rather bizarre suggestions in the name of science. I will not detail them in this book.

Certain people in the medical community – as well as many clinical psychologists – would like to suppress and outlaw the use of hypnosis by others, and gain legal control of its use for themselves. (Isn't this reminiscent of how the *elite* in ancient times sought to preserve the secrets of trance inductions?)

They created a gulf between the scientific community and the hypnotherapy profession, which I call the *Great Gulf.* A select few have tried to steal the livelihood of thousands of hypnotherapists by selling their opinions to lawmakers! This would cause the public to lose the power of choice while the *elite* dictated who could legally facilitate hypnosis.

There would be far more smokers in this country today if it weren't for the fact that hypnotherapy is a *legitimate profession.* Furthermore, many so-called "lay hypnotists" who practice *only* hypnotherapy have far more experience than other professionals who only use hypnosis occasionally.

Is the Great Gulf real?

So is there really a gulf between science and art? Some hypno-therapists have tried to convince me that this "gulf" between the artists and the scientists of hypnosis is only in my imagination, and cannot exist if I don't put any energy into it. But ignoring it won't make it go away. Unfortunate hypnotherapists in Texas tried ignoring this gulf, and woke up one morning in 1995 only to find that their livelihoods were suddenly legislated out of exist-ence! A well-trained or veteran hypnotherapist could not legally practice hypnotherapy in Texas; but a *mental health counselor* could use hypnosis even if he or she were only self-taught! *Is that fair?*

The A.S.C.H. has actively attacked the hypnotherapy profes-sion by claiming that hypnosis is "unprofessional" or dangerous unless done by someone with advanced degrees! This has been done through the media and in writing; yet many of those who criticize "lay" hypnotherapists actually received their training in hypnosis from members of the very group they attack.

In many ways this resembles the war between the A.M.A. and chi-ropractors, which has lasted for many years. But chiropractors are here to stay, as the public should have the freedom of alternative choices in health care. Chiropractors now control their own pro-fession – *as should we!*

Interestingly enough, the A.S.C.H. was not the first hypnosis asso-ciation to be born in this country. In Washington, a state associa-tion was founded in the early 1940s (the Washington Hypnosis Association). Also, the National Guild of Hypnotists (N.G.H.) was founded in 1951, pre-dating the A.S.C.H.; and there are increas-ing numbers from the scientific community bridging the gulf and affiliating with the N.G.H. and/or other hypnotherapy associa-tions that have formed through the years.

So do I give this gulf energy by being aware of it? My preference is to *put energy into building bridges across it!* One large hypnosis association has indicated in writing a policy of bridge-building; and I believe that more bridges MUST be built. Both the scien-tific community AND hypnotherapy must find ways to enhance communication and cooperation to bridge the gulf and keep hypnotherapy alive – for the sake of the countless numbers of people who need help!

Crossing the Great Gulf

There are many in the medical and academic communities who have already built bridges – becoming very accepting of well-trained hypnotherapists who might not have advanced degrees, wisely basing their opinions on the fact that *results speak louder than academic credentials!* I'll name a few ...

Donald Gibbons, Ph.D., was once a member of A.S.C.H. With a background as a clinical psychologist, he recognized the value of those called "lay hypnotists" who are competent enough to use hypnotherapy within the scope of their training and experience; thus he became involved in the hypnotherapy profession. He left the A.S.C.H. and joined a hypnotherapy association (The International Society of Professional Hypnosis), eventually becoming its executive director.

Another 20th century pioneer, Dr. Arthur Winkler, bridged the gulf by establishing a professional training program for hypnotherapists – without discriminating against those who lack advanced degrees. He obtained his Ph.D. in clinical psychology as well as a doctorate in theology, but then chose to become a hypnotherapist instead of a clinical psychologist. Before his passing, he hypnotized over 36,000 individual clients throughout his career, conducting much research with hypnotherapy, helping to bridge the gulf between medical hypnotherapists and the so-called "lay hypnotists" by teaching hypnotism to both physicians (and others who approach it as a science) as well as those who believe it to be an art. His widow, Pamela Winkler, Ph.D., worked closely with her husband. She also has a background as a psychologist – yet has done much to close the chasm between the scientists and the artists by promoting her late husband's programs.

Dr. Bernie Siegel, who has done wonders with hypnosis in the treatment of cancer, has gone so far as to recommend hypnotherapy in his book, *Love, Medicine & Miracles:*

> *A hypnotherapist can be valuable in the beginning, especially if the patient has trouble entering the state of deep relaxation. No matter who sets the course for the first meditative sessions – doctor, counselor, hypnotherapist, or the patient ... (p. 230)*

Dr. Siegel has helped bridge the gulf by evidencing public acceptance of hypnotherapy, both in his book and elsewhere. Dr. Irene Hickman, Dr. Edith Fiore, Dr. James Russell, Dr. Maurice Kougell, and numerous others have also helped to bring in an era of greater mutual acceptance and cooperation.

In addition, increasing numbers of physicians, psychiatrists and psychologists are referring some of their patients to hypnotherapists when hypnotherapy is indicated; and ethical hypnotherapists who know their limitations are referring clients back to other professionals when appropriate. Kevin Hogan, Ph.D., is a shining example of this cooperation; he specializes with patients who suffer from tinnitus, utilizing advanced hypnotherapy techniques with profound success. I highly recommend his book, *Tinnitus: Turning the Volume Down* (Network 3000 Publishing).

Where Is Hypnotherapy Today?

In the later decades of the 20th century, hypnotherapy finally came into its own and is now skyrocketing as a profession, thanks not only to people who span the great gulf like the Winklers and others mentioned above, but also to those who have worked almost exclusively in the training of professional hypnotherapists and / or creating professional hypnosis associations catering to the *full-time professional hypnotherapists.*

Charles Tebbetts became a living legend during his lifetime. He taught client-centered techniques, and also taught emphatically that all hypnosis is guided self-hypnosis – *truly making hypnosis an art.*

Also, names (in alphabetical order) like Harry Aarons (founder of the Association to Advance Ethical Hypnosis), Gil Boyne (American Council of Hypnotist Examiners), Dwight Damon (National Guild of Hypnotists), Tad James (author and internationally known trainer), Al Krasner (American Institute of Hypnotherapy), Sol Lewis (late hypnosis instructor with decades of experience), Ormond McGill (author of numerous books, and honored with the title of the Dean of Hypnosis), Anne Spencer (The International Medical Dental Hypnotherapy Association), and others, are likely to become legends in the history of hypnotherapy as a profession. Furthermore, people almost too numerous to list have promoted hypnotherapy without discrimination!

Numerous state and national professional hypnotherapy associations have sprung up in recent years – both in United States and internationally – promoting hypnotherapy as a career to people outside the medical community who wish to devote themselves *full-time* to the practice of the art.

Legal Recognition of Hypnotherapy

What I believe will go down in history as one of the biggest breakthroughs for the hypnotherapy profession came in 1987 in Washington State, when a state law was passed legally recognizing the hypnotherapy profession. This happened through the combined efforts of Charles Tebbetts, Fred Gilmore (a director of a state hypnosis association, the Washington Hypnosis Association), and a state senator at the time, Bill Kiskaddon, MSW – who was a certified hypnotherapist as well as a credentialed family and marriage counselor. The former Senator Kiskaddon also deserves a place in history for his work in getting hypnotherapy legally recognized in Washington State, as does Fred Gilmore.

Even though the United States Dictionary of Occupation Titles defines Hypnotherapist as a profession, the passage of Substitute

House Bill No. 129 in Washington accomplished three great benefits for hypnotherapy within the state: *first,* it provided some degree of public safety by requiring all hypnotherapists to register with the professional licensing division and adhere to the Uniform Disciplinary Code requiring certain professional ethics (discussed further in Chapter 9); *second,* this legal recognition helped hypnotherapy take a quantum leap within Washington. And finally, by early 1996, this recognition opened the door for insurance coverage; although some insurers fought it.

Other states have considered similar legislation – and it serves the public for hypnotherapy to remain *both legal and self-regulated* by the hypnotherapy profession. Just as chiropractors oppose regulation by physicians, neither do hypnotherapists wish to be regulated by psychologists.

Recognizing the credibility problems with the numerous 3-day and 5-day training programs, Indiana established a state certification requirement of 300 hours of training in order to practice as a Certified Hypnotherapist in that state.

The Future of Hypnosis

To help keep hypnotherapy legal, the *Hypnosis Motivation Institute* in California, founded in 1967 by Dr. John Kappas, obtained legislative assistance from the O.P.E.I.U. (an affiliate of the AFL/CIO). The *National Guild of Hypnotists* eventually jumped on board by forming Local 104, playing a key role in stopping detrimental legislation in Florida. Other hypnotherapy locals now exist. Also, a unifying organization was founded called the *Council of Professional Hypnosis Organizations* (C.O.P.H.O.) to create national acceptance of hypnotherapy, as well as to work with the Union to obtain legislation in numerous states ... with training requirements of around 100 hours. (While many feel 100 hours is low, at least it's a start!) The various hypnotherapy locals wish to promote greater professionalism of hypnotherapy as well as to help assure its legal survival and acceptance as a self-regulating profession, free of control by the psychology profession or by the A.M.A.

Thousands of hypnotherapists are involved in non-medical applications of hypnosis, as well as some medical applications under medical referral and/or supervision. Also, increasing numbers of people with medical backgrounds and other more advanced degrees are supporting the various professional hypnosis organizations; and they are all working to help promote hypnotherapy in a way that will finally bring it out of the dark ages once and for all.

In addition to all of the above, another modern day pioneer, Penny Dutton Raffa, founded the *International Hypnosis Hall of Fame*, an organization established to recognize people who make outstanding contributions to the field of hypnotism. Whether working as a scientist, or as an artist like Charles Tebbetts, those nominated by their peers and deemed worthy by a committee are honored. Mrs. Raffa believes that those honored today will be recognized as the historical pioneers of hypnotherapy tomorrow. Although the International Hypnosis Hall of Fame (IHHF) went into limbo after 2000 because of illness of the founder, a number of hypnotherapists hope that the IHHF will be revived someday.

The future of hypnosis finally looks bright – perhaps bright enough to grow and develop to its true full potential.

Chapter 4

The Dual Roles of Suggestibility Tests

Before we hypnotize anyone, we need to master a few mental exercises. This involves one or two simple "tests" of a person's ability to respond to suggestion and imagination. Such demonstrations prior to trance will help increase our chances of success. Most professionals call them *suggestibility tests*. (Some researchers prefer the term *waking suggestions*.)

Most hypnotherapy instructors, including my late mentor, have taught that the main objectives for suggestibility tests are *therapist* oriented: simply to test a client's ability to respond to suggestion as well as to determine the best techniques for hypnotic induction and deepening.

My professional experience successfully demonstrates to me that an even greater benefit in the use of suggestibility tests is actually *client oriented* – in helping sell the client on the fact that he/she can be hypnotized! (Charles Tebbetts eventually recognized the value in using these tests to help build a client's mental expectancy before hypnosis, but wrote it almost as a footnote at the very end of the subsection on suggestibility tests in Chapter 8 of *Miracles on Demand*.)

The way you ask a client to respond to any suggestibility test greatly influences the client's receptivity to hypnosis! *What* you say and *how you say it* strengthens the impact. Skilled and artistic use of such a test should build on all the ingredients of the hypnotic formula (belief, imagination, expectation and conviction), and help to replace a client's fear of hypnosis with comfort and confidence in both you and in the hypnotic process itself.

Wording is Important

What you say and how you say it will either increase or decrease your chances of success. Read this section carefully.

Before the suggestibility test

The best way to explain what you are doing with a client is to say:

I'm going to give you an opportunity to discover the power of your imagination ...

Why say it this way? First of all, from childhood up we all like to *find* things or *discover* things. (If desired, you may substitute the word *find* for the word *discover*.) Next, saying the words "the power of your imagination" makes the statement become *client-empowering*. The exercise demonstrates that it is *the client's own power* of imagination at work. Additionally, I tell my clients I'm going to "give" them something – and we like to be *given* to.

Do NOT say that you will test their ability to respond to suggestion, as has been recommended even in print by others. Some people have test anxiety (which can inhibit their comfort levels and possibly inhibit response), and using the word "test" in the explanation could push a panic button. Also, suggestibility is often equated with being gullible; so the phrase "suggestibility test" should only be used with other hypnotherapists.

After the suggestibility test(s)

Make full use of your client's response to a suggestibility test by saying:

> **Your fingers (or hands) did not move because I told them to –
> they moved because YOU imagined the magnets (or bucket).
> The power of hypnosis is in what you imagine. I'm only a
> guide – I can say the right words, but it is up to you to follow
> my instructions.**

By saying this, you have just helped your client appreciate the role of *imagination*. Furthermore, you have helped him/her *believe* that something will happen when it is imagined, because it already has! Then, if he/she follows your simple instructions as in the demonstration, the client can now *expect* something to happen. Why? As I tell all my clients:

Imagination is the language of the subconscious.

This is why hypnosis works. The subconscious does not know the difference between fact and fantasy, and responds to what is imagined just as though it is real.

Your words as a hypnotist should help the client use the imagination in a positive way, since the imagination is the *rehearsal room* of the mind. We can do anything we wish in our imaginations; and even though the conscious mind knows that it is not real, the subconscious reacts as though it IS real. Isn't that why we can cry in a good movie?

Now let's look at three suggestibility tests that Charles Tebbetts taught, updated with important variations ...

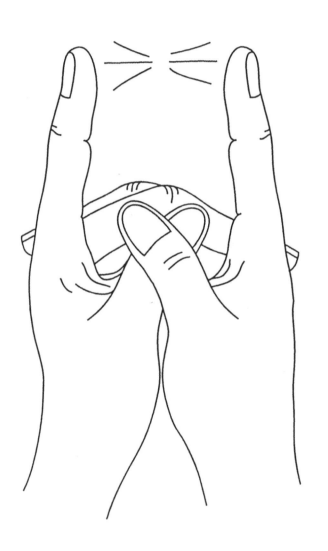

Tebbetts Suggestibility Tests (Roy Hunter style)

The Magnetic Fingers

This is my favorite, because it's fast, easy and effective.

> **I would like you to put both hands together and interlace your fingers. Now, straighten out both index fingers, and separate them about an inch. Now imagine a strong, irresistible force pulling your index fingers together as though you have magnets with opposite poles on your fingers. Now the magnets are twice as big, twice as strong.**

The moment they close, immediately explain to your client why the fingers moved (as explained previously). I often use two tests, so choose one of the next two (or skip this one and use both of the others).

Variation on Wolberg Arm Levitation

> **Stretch your arms out in front of you now, and close your eyes.**

Wait for response.

> **I am not going to hypnotize you quite yet. As I said, this is just a demonstration to help you find out how powerful your own imagination is, as well as to help me determine which hypnotic techniques best fit your personality.**

> **Imagine that I am tying a cord around your wrist ...**

Lightly touch client's wrist.

Imagine that a large balloon is tied to the other end of the cord, tugging your arm upward. SEE the balloon and FEEL it tugging.

Now, imagine that you're holding an empty bucket in your other hand, and I'm pouring water into the bucket. SEE the water pouring, HEAR the water splashing, and FEEL the bucket getting heavier as it gets fuller and fuller ... heavier and heavier ... pulling your arm down ... heavier and heavier, fuller and fuller ... as your other arm gets higher and higher.

When there is an obvious movement with one or both arms, stop the script and say:

Now, open your eyes and look at your arms.

There are numerous variables of this test. Mr. Tebbetts had clients imagine an iron dumbbell rather than a bucket. Wolberg used a weight. Some hypnotherapists ask clients to imagine a stack of books. Others prefer a bucket filling up with sand.

My preference for the water bucket is because people who are primarily auditory may easily imagine the *sound* of splashing water, yet they may be far less responsive to the other variations of this test.

Magnetic Hands

Charles Tebbetts frequently used the following technique, and openly gave credit to Gil Boyne for originating it. (Note that Charlie normally gave credit to others when appropriate, as he learned hypnotic tools from many people over the years. Some of my mentor's techniques are original.)

Now hold both of your arms out straight in front of you, elbows straight, fingers out straight, thumbs up.

Push his/her hands apart about 36 inches, then together, then about 24 inches apart. Then, place your index finger at a point halfway between client's hands.

Stare at my finger. I am going to count from three to one. At the count of one, close your eyelids down, and keep your eyes in the same position, staring at the spot where you last saw my finger ... three ... two ... one ... eyes closed.

Now, imagine that I am placing a magnet in the palm of this hand ...

Touch one of his/her hands.

... and now one with an opposite pole in your other hand.

Imagine the magnets drawing your hands together ... pulling and drawing, pulling and tugging ... feel the magnets tugging, closer and closer now ... closing now ...

When they touch, just let them drop into your lap, relax, and open your eyes.

True to the prediction of my former teacher and mentor, these three suggestibility tests are adequate for most of the people most of the time. In rare cases, I will ask a client, "Do you remember the sound of fingernails scraping on a blackboard?" and I will form my fingers into a claw shape. This will almost invariably get a response!

In case you wish to do your own research, numerous hypnosis books cover them adequately. Before his death, Charles Tebbetts gave a *very* high personal recommendation to *Hypnosis: the Induction of Conviction* by Dr. John C. Hughes (available from the National Guild of Hypnotists). The reader will find several excellent suggestibility tests to choose from in Chapter 10 of that book. Another, *General Techniques of Hypnotism* (by Andre Weitzenhoffer, Ph.D.), devotes two chapters to various suggestibility tests and variations (which he calls waking suggestions). These two books alone should give you enough suggestibility tests to last a lifetime if you wish to choose from a variety of them.

Should You Use Suggestibility Tests Every Time?

I recommend that you consistently use at least one or two suggestibility tests with *every first* session you have with a client, and more if needed. It is solely at your discretion to determine whether or not to use them with any subsequent sessions once rapport has been built and you know how well your client responds to the entire hypnotic process.

Before You Begin Hypnosis...

So now you've finished the suggestibility tests and you are ready to hypnotize your client. Now what? Charles Tebbetts required all his students to memorize the following words:

> **Are you ready to be hypnotized? All hypnosis is self-hypnosis. If you follow my simple instructions, no power on earth can keep you from being hypnotized. You can resist if you want to, but that is not why you are here. Just follow my simple instructions, and you are about to enjoy a very pleasant, relaxing experience.**

One of my students dubbed the previous paragraph as the "logo" during one of my classes, and that nickname quickly caught on and has stuck to this day with each successive class. Whenever I hypnotize a client for the first time, I will incorporate all of the above statements into my discussion prior to hypnosis; but I elaborate.

For example: I tell clients that if I suggest they imagine being in a peaceful place, but they imagine the freeway during the rush hour traffic, they won't be getting their money's worth. I then go on by asking, "If I suggest that you imagine being at your ideal weight, and you fantasize eating chocolate candy instead, what message will you be sending to your subconscious mind?"

I explain that I'm like a guide, a facilitator, or an *artist* who can say the right words, but it is up to each client to follow my simple instructions. Then I ask if they are ready to enter hypnosis.

The question, "Are you ready to be hypnotized?" is what I call the *magic question*. Why ask the magic question? The first time you are hypnotized *before you are ready* may help you to fully understand the answer – as I discovered once when I had to bring myself up out of deep hypnosis in order to use the facilities. Some people may have more questions. Others may wish to remove contact lenses, or kick off their shoes, etc., or step outside and have a smoke. And even if they are ready, failure to ask permission as you start could create slight resistance or resentment.

Now that both you and your client are ready, choose the hypnotic induction you prefer and *go for it!*

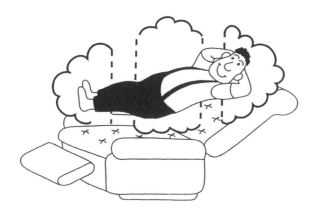

Chapter 5

Inductions and Awakening

Even though all hypnosis is guided self-hypnosis, the facilitator who masters basic hypnosis with competence and confidence endeavors to *make it easy for a client to follow suggestions.* This step begins by guiding the client into a trance; or, more accurately stated, the artist must effectively induce hypnosis! This is called a *hypnotic induction.*

Many researchers in the scientific community know numerous hypnotic techniques, as do many professionals in the artistic community. Although the average hypnotherapist may not need to memorize an encyclopedia of hypnotic inductions, it's very unwise to limit your knowledge of inductions. Many therapists using hypnosis have made the mistake of mastering only one or two induction techniques, resulting in their inability to help a client back into hypnosis if he/she awakens out of a deep trance. Unfortunately, there is no induction technique that works on all the people all the time; therefore it is imperative for the professional to master a variety of techniques in order to increase the probability of client success.

In other words, we must *fit the technique to the client rather than trying to fit the client to the technique.*

How Do We Induce Hypnosis?

Charles Tebbetts wrote in Chapter 8 of *Miracles on Demand:*

> *The moment the critical activity of the conscious mind slows down, the instant of passivity occurs. At this moment, the hypnotist gives the*

subject suggestions that cause him to bypass the critical factor and the trance state of hypnosis is achieved.

He continues to explain what he taught in Edmonds. All hypnotic inductions fall into six basic categories, or types; and every induction technique incorporates one or more of the six basic types. I call these the building blocks of all induction techniques.

When I studied at his school, Mr. Tebbetts taught us enough induction techniques to incorporate all of the six basic types. He furthermore wanted us to practice them enough to develop confidence and competence with all of them. Also, he described two hypnotic styles for inductions as well as all hypnotic techniques: *maternal* (gentle, permissive or lulling) and *paternal* (spoken with authority).

In my classes at Tacoma Community College, I teach my students enough techniques to develop skill with all of the six basic induction types as categorized by Mr. Tebbetts. Any master of the art of hypnosis, with an understanding of these six basic induction types, can blend them skillfully to create almost limitless induction techniques much the same as a painter can mix the three primary colors to create numerous shades of colors for the painting.

This chapter's objective is to provide both the student of hypnosis and the professional alike with the same information, and to present the techniques as I teach them at Tacoma Community College; but before you practice any induction type, make certain that you understand the section at the end of this chapter on awakening! If you wish, you may substitute the words *peace, relax* or *relaxation* instead of "sleep."

Editorial comments are in normal print.

What to say is in a bold print.

Instructions are in italics.

Induction Type #1: Eye Fixation

Hypnotic inductions portrayed by Hollywood often utilize some method of eye fixation. Any induction which has someone staring at a candle, gazing at a spot on the wall, or following a moving object such as a swinging pocket watch or spinning crystal or spiral, etc., is an example of eye fixation. The *fixed-gaze* inductions so popular in the 19th century were examples of eye fixation.

Charles Tebbetts taught that inductions depending *solely* on eye fixation or eye fascination have a higher than average failure rate. My personal experience validates this. Also, I fail to respond to eye fixation methods myself, as I am auditory and kinesthetic – but not very visual.

Perhaps some who have researched hypnosis scientifically and relied too much on eye fixation methods have mistakenly believed that some people are "insusceptible" because they resist eye fixation techniques the same way I do. (I can go very deep with some techniques and be unresponsive with others. Furthermore, since all hypnosis is self-hypnosis, *I have to want to be hypnotized*, otherwise I can easily resist.)

In my own classes those students who are not visual also seem to have the greatest difficulty responding to eye-fixation techniques. Mr. Tebbetts still, nonetheless, used to give his students an induction utilizing eye fixation along with eye-closure suggestions on their first night in Basic Hypnosis. He felt that every hypnotist should at least know how to use eye-fixation techniques for the benefit of clients who respond to them. With his permission (and his insistence), I have reproduced it verbatim for my professional hypnotherapy classes since 1987 – and have included it in this chapter. Out of respect for my former mentor, it is reproduced in the rest of this subsection *exactly* as Mr. and Mrs. Tebbetts gave it to me years ago (except "client" replaces "subject").

Charles Tebbetts Maternal Eye-Fixation Induction...

*Are you ready to be hypnotized?

*All hypnosis is self-hypnosis. If you follow my simple instructions, no power on earth can keep you from being hypnotized. You can resist if you want to, but that is not why you are here. Just follow my simple instructions, and you are about to enjoy a very pleasant, relaxing experience.

Your ability to become hypnotized depends largely upon your ability to focus your entire attention upon a small spot or object. In this case, the spot will be my (ring) (pen) (fingernail). Focus your eyes on my (ring) (pen) (fingernail) and don't let your eyes leave it for a single second.

Hold your hand about 12 inches from the client's eyes, raise it to a position where it causes a slight strain on his/her eyes (about 18 inches above eye level) each time you ask him/her to take the following deep breaths. Be certain you keep it within his or her range of vision. As the client exhales, lower your hand to its original position. Keep it in the raised position after the third breath.

All right, as you continue to stare at my (ring) (pen) (fingernail), take a long, deep breath and hold it in ... hold it in. Now let it all out and relax all over.

Lower your hand slowly.

SLEEP NOW. Take another long, deep breath. Hold it longer this time ... now let it all out and relax even more ...

Lower your hand again.

SLEEP NOW. Again, inhale, hold it in. I am going to keep my hand up this time. Keep staring at my (ring) (pen) (fingernail). Now, exhale ... and let a WAVE of relaxation go from the top of your head all the way down to the tips of your toes.

Keep your hand in a raised position.

I am going to count from five down to one. As I count, your eyelids become heavy, droopy, drowsy, and sleepy.

As you count, move your hand a little closer to the client's face and move it slowly downward. At number ONE, it will be six or eight inches below eye level.

Number five ... Eyelids heavy, droopy, drowsy, and sleepy.

Number four ... Heavier with every number you hear.

Three ... If your eyes go out of focus, that's all right. The next time you blink, that is hypnosis coming on.

Two ... Your tired eyelids want to close down. Closing, closing, closing down now.

One ... Now let your eyelids close down (if they have not already done so), and relax all over.

Always use at least one positive and beneficial suggestion while your client is hypnotized — such as one or more of the following examples:

You always enjoy the pleasant, relaxed feeling of hypnosis because your body becomes completely normalized when you relax.

Your glands work in harmony with one another; your body chemistry is perfectly balanced; and you feel good.

You also feel good when you come out of hypnosis – better than you have felt for years – not because I say so, but because your body is so completely normalized.

You feel good about yourself and you feel good about the world around you.

You feel great!

*HISTORICAL NOTE: Mr. and Mrs. Tebbetts required students to memorize the "magic question" as well as the asterisked paragraph following it, and say those words before any hypnotic induction. At their request, my students still have the same requirement. Chapter 4 explains how I weave those words into preparing my client for hypnosis. Review it if necessary.

Type #2: Relaxation (or Fatigue of Nervous System)

All induction techniques which simply have the client physically and mentally relax with his/her eyes closed use relaxation as one of the building blocks.

All progressive relaxation (or fractional relaxation) techniques fit into this category, as well as "guided imagery" or Ericksonian story-telling inductions requiring no physical response on the part of the client during the induction.

Charles Tebbetts referred to relaxation inductions as *fatigue of the nervous system*, and can be quoted as frequently saying, "This method usually bores the client into hypnosis." He believed that highly analytical people would generally resist this induction type on the first session. However, my own experience has proven that even analytical people can sometimes respond to a progressive relaxation type induction, provided they want to and it is done in an artistic way. A thorough explanation of hypnosis must be given ahead of time, as well as competent use of suggestibility tests to enhance belief, imagination, conviction and expectancy.

Successful use of an induction using relaxation alone, then, requires both client cooperation and artistic use of your voice (use vocal inflexion). As with any induction, remember to ask the "magic question" before you begin.

Here is what I say (pausing briefly at the dots ...):

The Roy Hunter Progressive Relaxation Induction

Whenever you're ready to begin, just close your eyes and take several deeeeep breaths ... and relax ...

Just take a journey of imagination, and imagine yourself in a safe, beautiful place of peace ... Imagine sights, sounds, and feelings that are so peaceful, so comfortable, and so relaxing, that it's easier and easier to relax with each breath you take ...

Notice how your thoughts can occur many times faster than the words of the spoken voice, so it makes no difference whether your conscious thoughts are listening, or drifting and wandering, or both, because your subconscious can respond to every word simply because you choose to allow it ...

So you are free to imagine more vividly such total tranquility that it becomes easy for you to become a part of the peace that you imagine ...

So just make it more real now by imagining a relaxation moving into your toes and your feet. And with each breath you take, it becomes easier and easier to go deeper and deeper relaxed ...

So just let this imaginary relaxation become more and more real as you move it through your ankles into your calves ... every nerve and muscle responding to your desire to relax ...

The relaxation just flows through your knees into your thighs, spreading up into your hips and stomach muscles ... circling your waist ... spreading up into your back... moving into the back of your shoulders and into the top of your shoulders, just as though gentle fingers have given you a soothing massage, and it just feels so relaxing that it's easier and easier to go deeper and deeper relaxed ...

Just let that relaxation spread up the back of your neck and into your scalp. And the more you imagine it, the more real it feels ...

Your forehead and temples relax ... Your cheeks and jaw muscles relax ... Every nerve and muscle relaxes completely ... And it feels so good to relax that it becomes easier and easier to go deeper and deeper as I count from ten to one ...

Beginning with Number 10 ... Deeper and deeper ... deeper into your imagination, imagining more vividly your place of peace ...

Number 9 ... Deeper and deeper ... your imagination is the rehearsal room of your mind ... where you are free to imagine total peace...

Number 8 ... Deeper and deeper ... relaxing physically ... deeper with each number ... and deeper responding to my voice ...

Number 7 ... Deeper and deeper ... relaxing mentally ... deeper with each number ... deeper because you choose ...

Number 6 ... Deeper and deeper ... relaxing emotionally. The deeper you go, the better you feel ...

Number 5 ... Deeper and deeper ... relaxing into hypnosis ... the deeper you go, the deeper you want to go, until I awaken you ...

Number 4 ... Deeper and deeper ... just relaxing completely ... the deeper you go, the easier it is to go even deeper ...

Number 3 ... Deeper and deeper ... into the rehearsal room of your mind ... imagining your place of total peace ...

Number 2 ... doubling the relaxation ... imagining sights, sounds, and feelings that are so relaxing that it's easier and easier to go deeper and deeper and deeper ...

Number 1, Waaaaaaaaay down deep ... into a very deep, hypnotic peace ... a very deep ... hypnotic peace.

Most everyone acquainted with hypnosis or meditation has heard a variation of progressive (or fractional) relaxation at one time or another. Also, it is a matter of personal preference whether you start from the feet up, or from the head down. (Notice that I say "peace" instead of *sleep*.)

Some hypnotists will end with relaxing the muscles in and around the eyes, using eye catalepsy as a hypnotic challenge or "convincer" for a deepening technique (refer to Chapter 7) rather than relaxing the jaw muscles last. Others will actually begin with relaxing the muscles in and around the eyes, and then use progressive relaxation throughout the rest of the body. I consider all of the above valid if done effectively.

As mentioned earlier, variations of relaxation inductions can incorporate *guided imagery*, which is frequently used by facilitators of group meditations. Often such meditations – whether used privately or in groups – rely heavily on visualizing, making the false assumption that everyone will find it easy to imagine *seeing* a stream or a beach, etc. If you facilitate such guided imagery, it's a good idea to find out first whether or not your client is visual, auditory, or kinesthetic, so that you may structure your guided imagery accordingly.

Charles Tebbetts normally asked people whether or not they could easily visualize. He also recommended that we ask our clients to describe their most peaceful place imaginable. This can be very helpful whenever guided imagery is used. Also, if you incorporate water, woods, or elevators, make sure they don't have any phobias of the above, etc.

If facilitating a group, include sights, sounds and feelings. For example, while a visual person could *visualize* the beach, an auditory person might find it much easier to imagine the *sound* of ocean waves – and someone who is kinesthetic would most likely *feel* the breeze and/or the sand beneath bare feet, and so on.

Type #3: Mental Confusion

Any technique designed to confuse the conscious mind can induce the hypnotic state once the critical faculty is bypassed, or the moment of passivity occurs. This type of induction is called mental confusion.

While the conscious mind keeps trying to find the logic in what is being said or done, the hypnotist gives suggestions to the subconscious mind to enter hypnosis and go deeper.

Charles Tebbetts taught two examples of mental confusion. I have incorporated my own style into his two techniques, and teach them to my hypnosis students.

The first involves instructing the client to close his/her eyes on even numbers and open them on odd numbers (or vice versa) as the hypnotist counts either forwards or backwards. As you start counting, watch for watering or redness in the whites of the eyes. When either of these begins, start pausing longer when the eyes are closed, and hastening when the eyes should be open. You may add words such as, "It becomes easy to forget, difficult to remember, whether your eyes should be open or closed... and as you forget to remember, or remember to forget, you just find yourself going deeper into hypnosis, or letting go totally..."

At the first sign of hesitation, start skipping numbers. This helps create more mental confusion, as in the first example:

Mental Confusion with Eye Closure

100, just close your eyes, take a deep breath, and relax ... You may notice the mind can think many times faster than the spoken voice, and that's OK ...

99, open them, take another deep breath, and 98 – eyes closed. Very good. Just imagine you're releasing all the cares of the day as easily as you release the air from your lungs ... 97, find it's getting more difficult to even try to open your eyes. 96, eyes closed. Good. Just find yourself wanting to go deeper and deeper as you forget whether your eyes should be open or closed, or closed or open ...

95, easy to forget. 94, difficult to remember, whether they should be closed ... and as soon as you forget to remember, or remember to forget, they stay closed, and you can just relax even deeper, or let go into hypnosis. 93, good! 92 ... deeper and deeper relaxed ... It's so easy to respond to my voice as I say 91, 90 ... your eyes just want to stay closed now.

Start speaking somewhat quicker and with more authority.

88, 86. Deeper and deeper. Easy to forget, difficult to remember, 84-82, whether they should be open or closed ... or is it closed or open ... 79, 75, 74. The numbers can skip away so quickly now that you just find yourself wanting to go deeper as your eyes want to stay closed. 72, 70. You can release yourself into deep hypnosis, or simply let go into total trance. 67, 65, 64. And every time you forget to remember, or remember to forget, open or closed, odd or even, you go deeper or deeper. 60, 50. Eyes closed and going deeper. Forgetting to remember, or remembering to

forget. 40, 30. Feeling good. Responding to my voice. Releasing, relaxing, letting go. Deeper and deeper.

Vary the numbers in the script according to how the client responds. Also, once your client leaves his/her eyes totally closed during an odd number, the moment of passivity has usually occurred. You may stop the counting if you wish and follow immediately with deepening suggestions (explained in Chapter 6), or continue on as part of the deepening.

In the above technique, Charles Tebbetts taught that you may enhance the mental confusion with incomplete sentences, or by bringing unrelated sentences and meaningless statements into the sleep and relaxation suggestions. (He gave Dr. Milton Erickson credit for this idea both in his class at Edmonds as well as in his book, *Miracles on Demand*.)

Mental Confusion with CLIENT Counting Out Loud

Another method of mental confusion taught by Charles Tebbetts involved having the *client* count out loud backwards from 200 or from 100, one number per breath, as well as the words "deeper" or "deeper asleep" after a short pause with each spoken number. You may then suggest that your client simply *"relax the numbers right out of your mind."* The client's conscious mind gets occupied with saying the numbers verbally while the subconscious is simultaneously hearing hypnotic suggestions. Talk in somewhat of a <u>monotone</u> as your client counts, pausing only briefly as he/she speaks each number. Use statements such as the following:

As you count, imagine you can see or hear the numbers before you try to find them, and they're getting farther and farther away. And I'll talk to your subconscious. You don't have to try to listen, just try to find each number. And as you skip numbers, repeat numbers, or forget numbers, you go deeper and deeper into hypnosis, or let go into a total trance. Just relax the numbers right out of your mind, allowing them to fade farther and farther, or smaller and smaller. Forgetting to remember, or remembering to forget. It's easier and easier to forget them or just relax them

away. Difficult to remember, or easy to forget. And the slightest hesitation between numbers DOUBLES your relaxation, or triples the trance ... sending you deeper into hypnosis, releasing, relaxing, and letting go ... you can either forget the last number, or the next number ... or the one before that ...

Once your client skips a number, the critical faculty is bypassed. Continue, while interjecting words such as ...

Very good. You're responding very good. Your conscious can either listen, or drift and wander, or both, while your subconscious is free to hear and respond to every word.

Notice the use of the word "good" rather than "well" in this statement. To some people, saying "well" might make them imagine a well in the ground. I learned this the hard way a few years ago after it took three sessions for me to successfully hypnotize a woman who had a phobia of wells. My professional opinion was validated by the late Arthur Winkler, Ph.D., (of St. John's University in Springfield, LA) who carefully researched the impact words have on the subconscious.

When your client stops counting, deepen immediately. Pay attention to your client's responses and adjust accordingly! If your client continues counting in sequence to the low 80s (or after struggling with a couple numbers), say some numbers yourself with words such as:

77. Double the hypnosis, or triple the trance ... 75, it's so easy to imagine whatever you wish as 74 causes your conscious mind to find it so difficult even to try to look for the numbers, that on 70, it's just easier to relax and forget to count, or simply go deeper. 64, 58. Very good. Perhaps the next number was 68 ... or was it 43? It makes no difference as the count goes below 30. You just find it easier and easier to respond to my voice as you go deeper and deeper on 25. Drifting right on down. You may be surprised at how deep you go, or perhaps you'll find yourself in total trance. You may even forget to remember the numbers I speak, or you can remember to forget where you stopped counting ... (etc.).

At this point, you may (if necessary) again enhance the mental confusion with more unrelated sentences and meaningless statements interjected with random numbers and suggestions for deep hypnosis.

While demonstrating this second technique to my class once, a student was determined to count all the way down in sequence to the number one; so when he got into the teens, I said, "When you say the last number, you are going deeper than you've ever gone before into *total hypnosis!*" He was still smiling on 2, but when he said the last number he slumped immediately into a very deep state of hypnosis.

Also, it's quite probable that the above technique evolved from a similar technique described by Dr. John Hughes as "John Hartland's Eye-Fixation with Distraction Induction" (pp. 74–75 of *Hypnosis: The Induction of Conviction*), which incorporates eye-fixation as well.

Type #4: Mental Misdirection

Mental misdirection is hypnotizing by conviction with use of any suggestibility test or a hypnotic "convincer" involving dramatic use of the imagination.

While mental confusion is designed to confuse the conscious mind until it is easier to just relax and let go, *mental misdirection* is any technique which incorporates a *physical response to something that is imagined.*

The only example of mental misdirection that Charles Tebbetts taught was a simple eye catalepsy technique which has the client close his/her eyes and roll the eyeballs upwards under closed eyelids, looking at an imaginary moon through an open window in the top of the forehead. Then the client is told it is impossible to open the eyes, and when he/she tries and fails, a feeling of hypnosis occurs. If the client successfully opens the eyes, then another technique should be used immediately without any conversation or obvious concern on your part.

My personal experience with this technique validates its effectiveness with most people who are visual; but I *neither* recommend it with people who are primarily auditory, nor with a client who has sensitive eyes. Because this technique gave me a headache when I experienced it, I created my own example of mental misdirection using a suggestibility test. My technique incorporates suggestions that one can respond to whether he/she is visual, auditory, or kinesthetic. It is reproduced here just as I teach it in my class at Tacoma.

The Water Bucket Induction

Ask client to extend both hands, palms up, and ask him/her to imagine holding an empty bucket in one hand, and helium balloons in the other. Also make sure you begin by asking the "magic question" as previously instructed.

Just close your eyes now and take a deep breath, and relax. Just IMAGINE that someone begins pouring water into the bucket, while someone else ties several dozen more helium balloons to the other hand.

Choose hypnosis, and you can be totally hypnotized when your hand touches your lap. But for now, just imagine that water is pouring into your bucket. SEE the water pouring into your bucket. HEAR the water pouring into your bucket. FEEL the bucket getting heavier and heavier. In fact, your arm begins to feel like it simply wants to drop right on into your lap so you can drop right on into hypnosis. Or you may feel your light arm getting lighter as the bucket gets heavier.

If the client's arm has reached his/her lap by now, <u>skip down to the double asterisk (**)</u>; otherwise, continue with the following, skipping down to the (**) <u>when the hand drops</u>.

That bucket is one-fourth full now. Every sound you hear just makes that bucket keep getting fuller. You can feel it getting heavier. SEE that water going in. HEAR it filling up your bucket.

It would be SO EASY to simply let your arm drop down into you lap so you can drop on into hypnosis.

Now take a deep breath and relax. As you do, notice your bucket is one-third full now ... and you have an increasing desire to let your arm drop. In fact, your arm may be feeling somewhat tired as you try to hold that bucket ... which is half full now. And the water just keeps pouring on in!

You feel an increasing desire to just drop that arm ... and when you do, you just drop right on into a pleasant hypnotic sleep ... releasing, relaxing, and letting go.

Even if the arm is still up, pay close attention to even the slightest downward movement, keying in on it. Vary your suggestions accordingly, using this script only as a guide.

As you notice your arm beginning to drop, that bucket is almost full now, and it is sooooo heavy!

The instant you start the next statement, touch the palm of the client's hand and speak very authoritatively ...

Somebody drops in a rock. SLEEP NOW!

** In a more soothing voice, continue with the following ...

The balloons are gone. Now just let both arms rest comfortably in your lap. Take a deep breath, and relax even deeper. It feels so relaxing, it's easier and easier to go deeper and deeper relaxed. In fact, every suggestion you accept helps you go deeper and deeper relaxed. Allow your arms to return to their normal weight. They feel totally comfortable now, completely rested and relaxed.

Continue deepening, using other suggestions as desired.

IMPORTANT: Give a suggestion for *normalizing both arms* to prevent any lingering effects after hypnosis! ALSO note that you should give this suggestion immediately after your client drops both arms into his/her lap, and then proceed directly to deepening techniques.

Type #5: Loss of Equilibrium

Mothers use this method to rock their children to sleep. This built-in desire to rock never seems to leave many of us, as is evidenced by the frequent desire to rock when some people sit in a rocking chair.

A few hypnotherapists use a rocking recliner, gently rocking their clients while they incorporate this induction type with progressive relaxation.

Charles Tebbetts did not teach any induction technique that incorporated only loss of equilibrium. He used this type as one of two building blocks for what he called the *rapid induction.*

Type #6: Shock to Nervous System

If a person imagines he/she can be hypnotized, believes he/she can be hypnotized, and expects to be hypnotized, and is convinced that you will induce hypnosis, then a *sudden surprise coupled with a command* given in an authoritative manner will usually result in instant hypnosis.

Charles Tebbetts taught two "rapid induction" techniques, which combined eye fixation, loss of equilibrium and shock to the nervous system. One of them (which I will not describe in detail) was what he called the "Gil Boyne" technique, which had the client *standing up* during the actual induction. At Charlie's request, I taught this when I first began teaching his course; but several years ago a professional hypnotherapist forgot to lock her knees when I demonstrated this to my class, and I picked her up off the floor amidst both laughter and concern from my students. I have since discarded this technique altogether.

The second technique can be useful in some circumstances in the office setting; and the few times I've used it in my practice, I've been very grateful for it. It is reproduced here exactly as written by Mr. Tebbetts (except that I've substituted the word "client" for the word "subject").

The Charles Tebbetts Rapid Induction

Sit with the client at your left (his/her right) with the front corners of your chairs touching.

If you can follow my simple directions, nothing outside yourself can keep you from becoming hypnotized. You can resist if you want to, but that's not why you're here.

I'm not going to hypnotize you yet, but I want to illustrate what I'm going to do. This will be a practice run.

Place your left hand behind the client's neck, and hold your right hand about two feet in front of his/her face.

Let's practice it now. I'm going to pull you forward, and when I do, bend at the waist and come forward so that your forehead rests in my right hand.

Pull the client GENTLY forward until his/her forehead rests in your palm. This establishes a muscular pattern. Straighten him/her back in the chair.

Now, are you ready to be hypnotized?

Wait for response!

Put your feet flat on the floor. Place your hands on your thighs and relax. Choose a spot on the wall ahead of you, and stare at that spot. Don't let your eyes leave it for a single second.

Place your left hand on the client's shoulder, rocking gently.

Want to be hypnotized, expect to be hypnotized, and you will be hypnotized.

Keep hand on the shoulder; continue to rock slightly.

Take a long, deep breath, and hold it in, hold it ...

Now let it all out, and relax all over.

Take another long, deep breath, and hold it longer this time ...

Now exhale, and allow your entire body to go loose and limp.

Now shift your left hand from the client's shoulder to the back of the neck.

As I count from five down to one, your eyelids become heavy, droopy, drowsy and sleepy. At the count of one, you go into a deep hypnotic sleep.

FIVE, eyelids heavy, droopy, drowsy and sleepy.

FOUR, heavier with every number you hear.

THREE, your tired eyelids want to close down now.

TWO, on the next number, allow your eyelids to close down completely and let every muscle and nerve in your body relax.

ONE ... SLEEP NOW!

Pull the client forward into your palm as rehearsed but more rapidly, and shout SLEEP NOW as he/she is moving between the original position and the position with his/her head in your palm:

Start to gently rotate the client's head the second it touches your palm. This keeps the subject slightly disoriented while you continue with another five-to-one countdown.

As I count from five down to one, you go deeper with every number you hear. Five, letting go more and more. Four, all of your cares and tensions are just fading away. Three, you are going deeper with every sound that you hear, and with every breath that you take. Two, just going deeper now. Deeper into a deep hypnotic sleep. Number one, just let go completely now, and be aware that you are bathed in the flow of a very pleasant, deep, hypnotic sleep. You hear my words at all times but remain in a deeeeeeep, hypnotic sleep, a deeeeeeep, hypnotic sleep.

Proceed immediately with another deepening technique.

SPECIAL NOTE: In a recliner, you may have the client sit straight up during the above induction and drop him/her back into the recliner instead of forward into your palm.

The above technique is considered to be paternal; but I have observed it done with similar wording in a maternal manner, with the emphasized command of "SLEEP NOW!" being the only paternal suggestion. I personally will only use this rapid induction method for a client who is resistant to most other inductions but has convinced me of a sincere desire to be hypnotized. I have also used this a few times with children who have short attention spans. And of course, I teach it to my students. It is effective, but I object to a hypnotist using this technique to serve his own ego.

One of my former students, a registered nurse, has frequently used the *Charles Tebbetts Rapid Induction* (as well as his own variation of a rapid induction) with hospital patients suffering in pain to help them get into hypnosis as quickly as possible for hypnotic pain management, with excellent results. Note that he only uses hypnotic pain management under supervision of a physician, or with an examining physician's written consent.

Paul Durbin, Ph.D., a hypnotherapist who worked many years in a New Orleans hospital, used a rapid induction involving a quick command spoken paternally the instant a set of keys strikes the floor. In another example, the patient holds a quarter (or one ounce of silver) in the palm of the hand, with the arm hanging slightly over the edge of the bed. Give suggestions to imagine the coin getting heavier and heavier, compounding with the suggestion for instant hypnosis when the coin drops (blending mental misdirection with the element of surprise).

Another rapid induction is a variation on the Elman technique, with the client pushing down on the palm of your hand while you count backwards from five to one, gradually increasing pressure as you count. Pull your hand out quickly on "two" with a command for instant trance (the client expects it to happen on "one").

Note that any rapid induction employed must be followed immediately with deepening techniques.

Unique Technique

In addition to the induction types described in this chapter, the use of *post-hypnotic suggestion* as an induction (explained further in Chapter 8) could be considered a *unique technique* that does not fit into any of the six basic types described in this chapter – thus making it virtually a seventh type of and by itself. We could also call it "sudden surprise" and categorize it as shock to the nervous system. Since I teach hypnosis more as an art rather than a science, it makes no difference to me how others categorize this rapid post-hypnotic induction technique. You decide.

IMPORTANT ADVICE REGARDING TOUCH

Many techniques of hypnosis taught by Charles Tebbetts involve the use of touch, which he frequently used without ever having repercussions; however I personally witnessed him asking permission when I studied at his school, as he knew that some people don't like to be touched.

Whenever you intend to use touch techniques at ANY time during hypnosis, ask permission before you ever begin the induction. The easiest way to ask, keeping it positive, is by saying, "Are you comfortable being touched?" If you begin the induction without asking that question, avoid the use of any touch techniques throughout the *entire* session!

Charles Tebbetts also emphasized the importance of making certain that you never touch in a way that could in any way be misconstrued as sensual.

Your Imagination is the Limit

When I give my students their practical exam, I ask them to skillfully demonstrate two different induction techniques just as they learn them in class. Once on their own, however, they can then create new ones or use other proven ones not taught in my class. These six basic induction types can be used in various combinations limited only by the imagination.

Many available books describe hypnotic inductions for those who wish to stick to established techniques. Among them is an excellent one by Myron Teitelbaum, M.D., J.D., entitled *Hypnosis Induction Technics*. I also highly recommend Dave Elman's book, *Hypnotherapy*, which contains some very important information for any serious student of hypnotherapy. Charles Tebbetts recommended Elman's book as well, along with *Hypnotism Today* by LeCron and Bordeaux (now out of print, according to Amazon.

com). Also a virtual "must" for the library of any practicing hypnotherapist today is *Hypnosis: The Induction of Conviction* by Dr. John C. Hughes (National Guild of Hypnotists). The availability of books continues to increase (visit my webpage at this URL: http://www.royhunter.com/bookreco.htm).

I can also add that my own experience of over a decade as a full-time hypnotherapist indicates to me that it is not necessary to be a scientific researcher of all of the proven techniques in order to successfully guide a client through hypnosis. Just be certain that you have enough techniques mastered to quickly and comfortably change techniques with clients who do not respond well to those you usually use. Your induction of choice should be considerate of the client.

VOICE: *Your Greatest Tool*

In virtually every hypnotic induction the hypnotherapist uses, voice is the single most important tool.

Some researchers advocate speaking in a monotone voice. While I sometimes deem it necessary to use a monotone, I normally vary my voice in pitch, emphasizing certain words with *feeling*. Since hypnosis is at least as much an art as it is a science, I believe that putting artistic feeling into your voice style can enhance the degree of client enjoyment as well as client responsiveness. This also increases appreciation of the trance experience. You can best accomplish this by becoming competent and confident with the techniques you have mastered, working intuitively from your "right" brain rather than by being an "operator" or "hypno-technician" who uses precision in an analytical way with hypnotic techniques.

It is a pleasure to observe a true artist guiding someone into the state of hypnosis; but it can be somewhat boring if it is just done in a mechanical way by someone trying to be perfect. In my opinion what some of our early hypnotic pioneers lacked in modern understanding, they made up for in their artistic styles. (Remember Mesmer!)

Just as music performed with precise accuracy can seem "empty" if done without feeling, so can hypnosis. At times when I have experienced hypnosis done with little or no artistic style, I have found myself getting bored and resistant even though wanting to go deeper – yet a true master of the *art* of hypnosis can guide me quickly into really deep states.

Some might wonder why I allow myself to be guided into hypnosis by another. I believe I'd be a hypocrite to the profession if I failed to take advantage of such powerful tools for change whenever I need help. Self-hypnosis is like a muscle: I can easily lift a chair, but a couch is much easier to move with someone else helping me lift.

Also, I use the tools to help teach the tools. My students must practice being both the hypnotherapist and the client in the learning process, with suggestions to master the art.

If you are already using hypnosis, but wish to become a better artist, consider setting aside your pride and asking another hypotherapist to use the tools to help you master the tools. Even students of the legendary Milton Erickson experienced hypnosis, according to what Ronald A. Havens wrote on page 237 in *The Wisdom of Milton H. Erickson: Hypnosis & Hypnotherapy* ...

> *When Erickson sought to train hypnotherapists he did not just lecture them, he hypnotized them. There are several possible explanations for this. First, because experience is the best teacher, it makes sense to experience what it is you wish to learn. Secondly, because the hypnotist is basically attempting to teach the subject how to experience a particular set of internal events, it is reasonable to believe that the teacher should have learned to experience those events also. It is often difficult for someone who has never participated in a particular endeavor to teach others how to do it.*

Amen! Re-read that last statement. But now, before we even *consider* guiding anyone into hypnosis, we need to know how to awaken someone properly from the trance state.

Awakening

The sample script for awakening is placed on purpose at the end of this chapter so that it will be easy to find. But first, some words of advice are important for both the novice and the veteran alike... Avoid sudden or abrupt awakenings except in dire emergency, as your client may feel the same way you or I feel if suddenly awakened from a nap. The result of awakening too quickly could be momentary dizziness and/or a slight headache. I call this "hypnotic hangover."

My recommendation is a minimum of *at least* 30 to 45 seconds. I frequently take twice that long – and sometimes even a little longer for someone in a very deep state. Also, to increase response probability, raise your pitch or volume and slightly increase your tempo. If awakening is done in a monologue, a client in a deep state may not respond.

Counting is also important. If you count backwards for inductions and/or deepening, count forward to awaken (as in the script below). If you choose to count forward for inductions and/or deepening, then reverse the direction on the awakening suggestions. Failure to do this could result in the client going deeper instead of awakening. And the best way for you to remember which way you should count is to choose your preference and be consistent!

The script for awakening presented here is reproduced verbatim as Mr. Tebbetts wrote it, except for the last phrase of "Three..." (about driving alertly) which I added in 1988. It is an excellent awakening script for most non-therapeutic uses of hypnosis. For hypnotherapy, you might wish to consider adding some additional positive suggestions.

The Charles Tebbetts Awakening Script

Now, I am going to count from one up to five and then I am going to say "fully aware." At the count of five, let your eyelids open and you are calm, refreshed, relaxed, fully aware, and normal in every way.

One ... Slowly, calmly, easily, and gently you are returning to your full awareness once again.

Two ... Each muscle and nerve in your body is loose, limp, and relaxed – and you feel wonderfully good.

Three ... From head to toe you are feeling perfect in every way ... physically perfect, mentally alert, and emotionally serene ... and when you get behind the wheel of your vehicle, you are totally alert in every way, responding appropriately to any and all traffic situations.

Number four. Your eyes begin to feel sparkling clear, just as though they were bathed in fresh spring water. On the next number now, let your eyelids open and you are then calm, rested, refreshed, fully aware, and feeling good in every way.

Number five, eyelids open now. You are fully aware once again. Take a deep breath, fill up your lungs, and stretch.

For the new student, practice at least one of these inductions and the awakening script before you go deeper into this book. *(NOTE: If you plan on using hypnosis professionally, seek competent training!)* Once you feel a level of confidence with at least one of the induction techniques, then you can learn the deepening techniques. However, I suggest that you choose at least one mental confusion technique to master, along with the mental misdirection technique described. It's also wise to eventually master a relaxation induction as well as one rapid induction. Then practice, *practice, PRACTICE!*

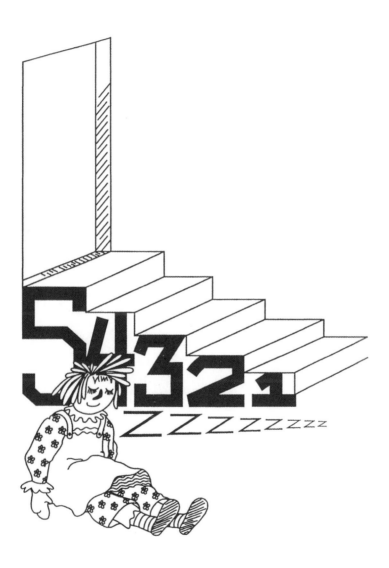

Chapter 6

Deepening the Hypnotic State

After you induce hypnosis, it is usually necessary to guide your client deeper into the hypnotic state to help validate the experience as well as to minimize the likelihood of him or her coming up to full consciousness too soon.

Recognizing the Trance State

A person in hypnosis becomes very relaxed, and usually evidences slow diaphragm breathing. The pulse rate normally slows down and there may be eye moisture or redness in the whites of the eyes. There may be fluttering of the eyelids, and/or rapid eye movement; or the eyeballs may roll upward. The face relaxes into an expressionless appearance which many people call the "hypnotic mask." Usually a client entering hypnosis will expel air in a long, deep breath, often referred to as the "hypnotic sigh."

The hypnotized person then usually becomes highly responsive to suggestion and direction; and even though he/she can be selective in the suggestions responded to, acceptance is usual – and frequently automatic – unless there is an emotional desire to resist. This "automatic" response, often the result of *compounding suggestions*, is perhaps why so many people have erroneously assumed that the hypnotist is in control of the person's mind.

There are various depth levels of hypnosis, each with its normally accompanying signs. Not all of these signs will occur – and some may occur at levels other than normal – but they are all common signs indicating at least a light trance state has been reached.

Let's discuss the various signs of hypnosis, along with the various trance levels, before looking at some actual deepening techniques.

Depths of Hypnosis

Opinions vary about how many depth levels of hypnosis there are as well as what constitutes evidence of each level.

Remember our discussion of Dr. James Martin Charcot in Chapter 3? He and the pupils at his academy succeeded in proving that there were several stages of hypnosis, and that a hypnotized person is capable of showing different symptoms and passing different "tests" in each stage.

Charcot's names and definitions of the three basic depths of hypnosis became acceptable standards that survive to this day. Various hypnotists use other scales composing four, five, seven, or more stages of trance depth, but the three-step scale devised by Charcot continues to be the most practical. The names that Charcot applied to the stages, in order, are *LETHARGY*, *CATALEPSY*, and *SOMNAMBULISM*.

These are often simply called (in the same order) light, medium, and deep. Even other scales include these basic levels, such as the famous Davis-Husband scale of hypnotic depths, the LeCron-Bordeaux scale, and so on.

Although Charles Tebbetts agreed with Charcot's three widely accepted levels, he based his descriptions of the various levels of hypnosis loosely on the LeCron-Bordeaux system for indicating depth levels of hypnosis. (The depth levels and signs are detailed in the book, *Hypnotism Today*, by LeCron and Bordeaux.) He included the *hypnoidal stage* (a very light state) in his descriptions of the states of hypnosis in his class as well as in his book, *Miracles on Demand*.

The *hypnoidal* stage is considered to be evidenced by a great deal of physical relaxation where the eyes close and often flutter for a while. There is partial lethargy of the mind, and the limbs may feel heavy to the person experiencing this stage. I rarely mention this state to clients, as I prefer to consider this a part of the light state.

Light

The light (or *lethargic*) state person evidences a great deal of physical relaxation, breathing more slowly. He/she may feel heaviness or lightness throughout the body, as well as an increasing disinclination to move, speak or think. (Some refer to this as partial lethargy of the mind.) There is also an *increase* in awareness of anything perceived through the five senses, so an analytical client may be much more aware of background noises, or garlic or alcohol on the breath! There can be catalepsy of the eyes and limbs, inhibition of small muscle groups, as well as greater response to suggestions.

Medium

In a medium trance state (also called the *cataleptic state*), one may respond to illusion suggestions, such as seeing something that is not real, or failing to see something that is real. The medium state client may be able to attain kinesthetic illusions (complete muscular inhibitions, such as inability to bend an arm), partial amnesia and glove anesthesia (numbing of the hand so that no pain is felt), and a firm conviction that he/she is in the trance state – although some people might find it difficult to describe.

Deep

In the deep or *somnambulistic* state, one has the ability to open his/her eyes without affecting the level of trance, and may experience uncontrolled movement of the eyeballs as well as profound sensations of lightness or floating. The pupils may be dilated. Complete hypnotic amnesia may occur, as well as amnesia of post-hypnotic suggestions that, if accepted, may still be carried out after trance termination. During somnambulism, the client may experience all types of illusions including vivid ones, and may even have an illusion continue for a limited time after leaving hypnosis. He/she may control the involuntary functions of the body such as heart rate, blood pressure and digestion. (Be careful, however, to avoid giving medical suggestions unless you are either licensed to do so or are specifically authorized by an examining physician!) This is the best state for certain hypnotherapy techniques described in Part II of this work, such as age regression and for recalling lost memories, as well as the effective parts therapy techniques made legendary by Charles Tebbetts.

Beyond somnambulism...

Dave Elman described an even deeper state in his book *Hypnotherapy* (Westwood Publishing), which he called the *Esdaile state*. In Chapter 13 he provides interesting historical background, including detailed instructions for inducing the Esdaile state as well as bringing someone back.

This state was named after Dr. James Esdaile, a 19th century physician, who performed surgery in India using this very ultra-deep state of hypnosis to anesthetize his patients. (Some professionals use other names for this state.)

The hypnotized person who attains the Esdaile state will hear all of your suggestions, but feels too lazy to respond to any of them. If you have clients enter this state, you may find them resisting your suggestion to awaken. If this occurs, use a much longer awakening count. Tell them as you begin counting that if they ever want to go this depth again, enjoying the peace, comfort, security, and recall that goes with it, it will be IMPERATIVE to awaken. Then dramatically increase your voice volume, speed and pitch as you count.

According to Elman, one out of several thousand people will spontaneously go into this ultra-deep state. After two years in my hypnotherapy practice, this happened to one of my clients during the latter part of a session. When she failed the second time to respond to my awakening instructions, I touched her hand and loudly said, "It's time to wake up!" Her face remained in the hypnotic mask, and she snored. Fortunately I remembered Elman's instructions as summarized above, and was relieved when it worked! She told me that she heard every word, but had no feeling whatsoever in her body other than a total euphoria – and absolutely did not want to come back just yet. However, she said she *knew* she had to come back when I told her that she could never go that deep again if she resisted waking up.

Charles Tebbetts did not write of the *Esdaile* state in his textbook, but he discussed it in his classes at Edmonds. I sometimes demonstrate this state to my own students.

LeCron and Bordeaux defined the ultra-deep level of hypnosis as *plenary trance*, where one experiences a stuporous condition in which all spontaneous activity is inhibited. It has also been called the *coma* state by many professionals, including Walter Sichort, who demonstrated this state at national hypnosis conventions in front of many hypnotherapists nationwide.

Mr. Sichort, who also taught hypnosis to many physicians throughout the country, believed that there are ultra-deep states even deeper than plenary trance. And indeed, I saw him demonstrate a state so deep in New York back in 1989 that when the volunteer accidentally fell off the chair and struck his head sharply on the corner of the podium, he did not even move a muscle! Then, with a few well-formulated post-hypnotic suggestions from Mr. Sichort, not only did the volunteer emerge from hypnosis without a bump, he also had no conscious memory of even striking his head!

Whether this man was in a plenary trance, coma state, Esdaile state – or an even deeper state – is still a matter of opinion. Again let me state that opinions vary about the number of levels of hypnosis, as it is *subjective rather than objective*. I saw one chart several years ago which actually subdivided the depths of hypnosis into over 20 levels. Charles Tebbetts felt that most people prefer to have everything labeled and neatly placed in orderly categories and indicated onto charts; but he also believed this tended to trap people into avoiding the fact that there are always exceptions.

Unless you are conducting scientific research in hypnosis, you can simply decide which method(s) of defining depth levels you like best and act accordingly. With experience, you may discover a great ability to recognize the depth of trance by the quality of response by your clients.

I believe, as my former mentor did, that the *results of the suggestions given* are much more important than trying to accurately measure the depth of trance obtained. This is especially true for any artist of hypnosis practicing client-centered hypnotherapy; although many medical applications of hypnosis may require that the patient be at least in a somnambulistic state for best results – necessitating a greater ability for the hypnotist to more accurately measure depth.

Some books charting hypnotic depths rate a certain percentage of people as "insusceptible" to hypnosis. If there is total client resistance without any apparent reason, it does not necessarily mean your client is actually "insusceptible."

Although total unresponsiveness might be due to either lack of artistic competency of the hypnotist, and/or lack of understanding on the part of the client (which may or may not be the result of improper pre-hypnotic discussion), and/or lack of trust or rapport, or simply because of how the client *feels* on the particular day, there is also another unpleasant possibility: your prospective client might be the victim of a "hypnotic seal" placed by another hypnotist who did not want anyone else to hypnotize him/her. Worse, he/she might not even remember having received such a disempowering suggestion! This very unethical practice is discussed in Chapter 9 of this book, along with a potential way to reverse the damage.

How to Deepen the Hypnotic State

The rest of this chapter is written to present and explain the deepening techniques taught by Charles Tebbetts.

Counting down (or up)

Suggest to clients that as you count backwards from five to one (or ten to one) that each number helps them go deeper and deeper.

FIVE ... you are going deeper with each number, relaxing completely. FOUR ... deeper and deeper, relaxing into hypnosis. THREE ... deeper and deeper, going deeper with each number. TWO ... deeper and deeper, into pleasant hypnotic relaxation. ONE ... just drifting down, down, down, Waaaaaaaay down, deeper and deeper relaxed.

Floppy arm (Dave Elman technique)

My mentor gave Dave Elman credit for this technique. (For those interested, Gerald Kein of Omni Hypnosis in Florida continues the work of the late Dave Elman.) Pick up client's arm by thumb (at the palm) or wrist, moving it back and forth while saying:

Just let your arm become limp and loose. Imagine it feels like a wet dishrag (or wet noodle)... limp and loose, just like a wet dishrag (or wet noodle). When I drop your arm into your lap, just let yourself go TEN TIMES DEEPER!

Drop client's arm as he/she exhales, and immediately say:

Now go TEN TIMES DEEPER.

If client tries to help you by lifting his/her arm, move it up and down as well as back and forth, and emphasize letting it feel totally like a wet dishrag, saying:

Just let me have the full weight of your arm ... and when I drop your arm into your lap, just let it flop down like a wet dishrag (or wet noodle) and go TEN TIMES DEEPER.

REPEAT with other arm. When using this technique, pick up client's hand either by the wrist, or by the thumb, grasping part of the palm to prevent discomfort. If possible, drop arm as client exhales.

Deepening by re-induction

Eye fixation example (taught by Charles Tebbetts):

When I ask you to open your eyes, I want you to look at my ring, keeping your eyes FIXED on my ring (pen, pencil, etc.). And I would like to establish a signal between us, that whenever I snap my fingers and say the words "SLEEP NOW!" you just close your eyes again and go even DEEPER into hypnosis. Now, open your eyes and look at my ring.

Hold your ring (pen, pencil, fingernail, etc.) about 12 to 18 inches from client's eyes, moving it up about 45 degrees above their plane of vision. Move it down below the plane of vision while saying:

As you watch my ring, your eyes just feel like closing – so (*snap your fingers*) SLEEP NOW! Just take a deep breath and go ten times deeper.

Pause just long enough for client to take a deep breath, and then continue:

Each time I ask you to open your eyes, it takes more effort – and you have an increasing desire to close them again. Now, open your eyes again and look at my ring.

Repeat above process several times, watching for eye fatigue, watering, etc.

NOTE that you may use almost any effective induction technique as a deepening technique – thus, Charles Tebbetts taught that the repertoire of your deepening techniques is at least as large as your repertoire of induction techniques.

Pushing gently on shoulders

Charles Tebbetts called this the *shoulder push* technique.

Explain to client:

As I step behind you and gently push down on your shoulders, I want you to go much deeper relaxed.

Step behind client, placing your hands gently on the shoulders. Do not push down until he/she exhales! Continue...

Now take a deep breath ... hold it in ... Now let it go ... (*Push down as he/she exhales.*) **Now go even deeper than before!**

Do this three times, resting your hands lightly on the shoulder between each push.

In the above technique it is important that you keep your hands *still* between pushes. Massaging the back or shoulders may either feel threatening to the client, or it may feel so good that he/she would want you to continue – distracting from the purpose of the hypnosis. Also, to avoid any possible misperceptions, *caution* must be exercised with the use of this technique with a member of the opposite sex!

Arm levitation with both direct and indirect suggestion

Charles Tebbetts taught this technique in my class back in 1983. I believe it to be a variation of a similar technique he borrowed from a videotape of Dr. Milton Erickson which he showed to my hypnotherapy class back then:

> **If you want to go deeper into relaxation you can feel even better as you raise your arm higher and higher. Each movement of your arm upward causes your whole body to go deeper and deeper into relaxation. Your whole arm becomes lighter and lighter, just as light as a feather floating in the breeze, and if you really want to go deeper into relaxation you can allow your arm to rise. Every motion of your arm upward causes you to enjoy a wonderful feeling of comfort. With each tiny motion of your arm rising upward, you will say to yourself, "I am relaxing even more." Just feel yourself going deeper with every breath that you take, with every beat of your heart, going deeper, or simply letting go totally.**

> *Give the client about 30 seconds of silence several times during this procedure. After the arm is extended upward at a right angle to his/her body, say:*

> **Now you are much deeper in hypnosis than you were a few moments ago. I am going to count to three, and at the count of three your arm will drop to your side (or lap). The moment it drops, you can go ten times deeper relaxed. One ... two ... three ... TEN times deeper relaxed.**

Frequent suggestion

In addition to using specific suggestive techniques for deepening the level of hypnosis, the hypnotist may also employ the frequent use of direct and indirect suggestion for the client to go deeper, such as in the following examples:

> **Choose a deeper state of hypnosis, DESIRE a deeper state of hypnosis, and you WILL go deeper with each suggestion you accept.**

Take a deep breath, relax, and go much deeper, or let go.

You can go deeper and deeper now, or find yourself surprised when you let yourself go into total hypnosis.

Every suggestion you accept takes you deeper and deeper, or more completely into a state of hypnotic peace.

The deeper you go, the better you feel.

It's so enjoyable to let go completely, deeper into peace.

Your conscious mind can relax completely, and your subconscious mind is free ... to respond to my voice.

The sound of my voice can take you deeper and deeper until I awaken you.

The deeper you go, the deeper you want to go, or you can simply release yourself into total trance.

Your entire body is responding to the idea of relaxation.

Being hypnotized is always a very pleasant, very enjoyable, soothing, restful, deeply relaxing experience.

It's so easy to respond to my voice ...

... releasing, relaxing, and letting go.

And so on ...

What about Guided Imagery for Deepening?

Numerous techniques incorporate guided imagery and/or programmed imagery for deepening, such as walking down stairs,
going down an escalator or elevator, etc. While all the above (or
variations) may be very effective with some people, nothing will
work with all of the people all of the time.

One of my personal favorites is to imagine myself going down an
elevator. Since imagining the downward movement is very effective for me, I incorporated the elevator with counting down when
I first began professional hypnosis. Then, within just a few weeks
of practice, a woman who had gone rather quickly and easily into
hypnosis terminated her trance suddenly with the words, *"I hate
elevators!"* After several unsuccessful attempts to regain rapport, I
refunded her money and referred her elsewhere. So you might say
I made a financial investment in the realization that it is wise to ask
your client about elevators (or steps, woods, water, lights, the sky,
or the country, etc.) *before* incorporating them into guided imagery
– as some people have phobic reactions to places and things that
others might enjoy totally.

I've also been on the *resisting* end of deepening techniques that
incorporate *going down stairs*. Why? Because I go down a flight of
stairs in seconds rather than minutes. While the hypnotist asks me
to go down the first step and look around, I go all the way to the
bottom and wait impatiently for the next deepening technique. In
the first place, I'm not very visual – so I do *not* stop to look around.
Secondly, if too much time is taken before the facilitator gets where
I already am, my own trance state is history. Yet I know people who
respond quite well to the guided imagery of going down stairs as
a deepener.

Charles Tebbetts once used a brief imagery of a trail in the woods
with forest sounds, and I really identified with it. Expanding on his
technique, I combined it with mental confusion by having the client
look for numbers like on a self-guided nature trail; only some of the
numbers are missing. By incorporating a stream, a waterfall, wild-
flowers, birds singing in the trees, a gentle breeze, etc., it becomes

a pleasant journey into the *woods of deep hypnotic peace.* Whenever I use this, however, I make certain my client *likes* the woods!

Again, as with any hypnotic technique, use only those deepening techniques you would be comfortable responding to if you were in your client's shoes. Balance your decision with the awareness that your client's likes and dislikes may *differ* from your own. One of my students failed to do this in class one time, and used a programmed imagery of a gentle rocking in a rowboat as a deepening technique. The client suddenly brought himself out of hypnosis and blurted out loud, *"I'm sea-sick!"* and bolted for the door. You can guess the rest of the story.

Whenever possible, ask another hypnotist to use a technique on you if you wish to try it out on others. Also, if you have read this far without ever being on the receiving end of hypnosis, I now urge you to experience it for yourself, with a trained and certified hypnotherapist.

Although a scientist researching hypnosis need not necessarily experience that state (nor a licensed physician using medical applications of hypnosis), I believe that all full-time professional hypnotherapists must experience hypnosis in order to be completely effective and true to the profession.

To be a good artist, you must experience the art on both the giving and receiving side! A neurologist in my class was just as willing to allow other students to hypnotize him as he was to hypnotize other students in the class; and he even asked them to call him by his first name. His attitude was a credit to the medical profession.

If you are afraid to let someone else guide you into the state of hypnosis, perhaps you might be well-advised to find out why, and then deal with your own resistance. If your resistance to being hypnotized is because you believe that someone else will "control" your mind, then it is my strong opinion that you have no business EVER hypnotizing others!

Whether you are already a professional hypnotherapist, or a student of hypnosis, or simply a curious reader who picked up my book, please EXPERIENCE the state of hypnosis if you ever intend to hypnotize anyone else. You owe it both to yourself and to all the people you guide into hypnosis!

Chapter 7

Testing During Hypnosis

Some researchers of hypnosis have used hypnotic testing as a means of "testing" their subjects for trance depth. Often they are called "challenge suggestions" because they are given to help the person in hypnosis go deeper into the state after acceptance of the challenge suggestion. They also help the hypnotist to estimate trance depth.

However, as with suggestibility tests, there is another very important *client-centered* benefit in giving this type of suggestion. Charles Tebbetts recognized this fact, and commonly referred to these "challenge" suggestions as hypnotic "convincers" because they helped convince a client that he/she really was experiencing hypnosis.

How Does Testing Benefit the Client?

Most people entering hypnosis for the first time often fail to recognize the hypnotic state because of common misconceptions. They know where they are, and hear everything you say; and because they know they could leave any time they wish, they frequently have difficulty accepting the fact that they actually have entered hypnosis.

As mentioned above, each "convincer" a client accepts helps deepen the state of hypnosis and helps to validate his/her trance experience. Furthermore, as the scientific community discovered, testing gives the hypnotist an indication of trance depth – which is important information for both the hypnotherapist and client alike before proceeding from the hypnotic techniques into hypnotherapy techniques.

Six techniques are presented in this chapter; four are presented just as taught by Charles Tebbetts (except where noted) – and the fifth and sixth are variations on arm levitation that I frequently use with my clients. As with other basic techniques, the actual number of hypnotic tests is limited only by your own imagination; but please give only suggestions that you would comfortably accept in a role reversal.

Eye Catalepsy Test

Mr. Tebbetts normally used this common "convincer" first, because it only involves small muscles that control the eyelids. Tell the client that as you count from five down to one, his/her eyelids are locking tighter and tighter.

> **Now that your eyelids are closed down, you'll find them locking themselves tightly shut. As I count from five down to one, just find them locking tighter with every number.**

> *Some therapists (including Mr. Tebbetts) have enhanced client-response by touching the person's hairline at the center of the forehead at this point – and then, while counting, moving one or more fingers slowly down, finishing at the bridge of the nose on number one. (I personally do not incorporate touch with this technique; but I felt it would honor my former teacher to mention how he added the element of touch.)*

> **FIVE ... the eyelids are beginning to lock tighter now. FOUR ... they are locking tighter with each number. THREE ... lock them even tighter now. TWO ... imagine they are glued shut! ONE ... they are locked so tight that even if you TRY to open them you FIND that they just lock tighter and tighter. Try to TEST them and find the harder you try, the more you find they just want to stay shut ... Now just relax all those muscles that control**

your eyelids. In fact, just relax all over and go even deeper into hypnosis.

Mr. Tebbetts taught that the use of the words "try" and "find" are very important in helping a client respond to any hypnotic "convincer" or test. The word "try" implies failure to the subconscious; so when you precede a suggestion with "try" the implication is that it will be difficult or impossible. Use of the word "find" is also important, because it is a positive word. Children love to "find" things; and that includes the child-like quality all of us have inside our own subconscious minds. Furthermore, since some people don't like "tests," some clients may not even try to "test" their eyelids. The late Arthur Winkler took advantage of that fact by using different language with the eye closure test:

Test them and make sure they remain shut.

I like *adding* the above statement whenever I use this test. (Note: use of the word "test" is OK for a convincer.)

The Hand Clasp

Ask client to put the palms of his/her hands together, lacing and interlocking the fingers together. Say paternally:

Imagine your fingers are like heavy, metal springs or vice-grips locking tighter together as I count from one to three. ONE, locking tighter with each number. TWO, lock them tighter and tighter now, like vice-grips. THREE, locking so tight that if you TRY to pull them apart, you FIND they just lock tighter and tighter. Test them and find they just lock tighter and tighter.

Pause only two or three seconds, and then grasp his/her hands at the wrist; and then continue maternally ...

THREE, TWO, ONE ... RELAX your hands, and simply allow me to gently pull them apart for you. Now take a deep breath and go MUCH deeper.

In the above example, it is important that your pause be *only two or three seconds* in order to minimize client discomfort and/or reduce the possibility of your client actually pulling his/her hands apart. Watch the hands *closely* during the short pause; and if you suspect that your client might pull them apart, then quickly suggest that they can be pulled apart. Then, without talking about it, go right on to another test.

When Charles Tebbetts used the hand clasp test, he had his clients stretch out their arms, and suggested that they then stiffen them and lock their elbows – squeezing the fingers against the backs of their hands. Then he suggested that they imagine *both hands and arms were one block of wood*. He still used the words "try" and "find" with this test. Also, when his client responded to this convincer, he would grasp his client with both hands at the wrists and push his thumbs against the pulse while suggesting that the hands *come apart with ease*. He would then pull the hands apart, dropping them into the client's lap as an additional deepening technique.

My personal experience has shown client results to be virtually as good without asking the client to lock the elbows as my teacher did; but you are free to make your own choice.

The Rigid Arm Test

Pick up client's arm and place it in a vertical position above his/her head. (This is where they lock the elbow!)

Lock your elbow, clench your fist, and reach for the sky ... (or ceiling)

Squeeze the arm at the elbow, forearm, wrist, and above as you continue...

Let all of the energy go up into your arm. Make it as stiff and rigid as a steel bar. Just as stiff and rigid as a steel bar. Your elbow is locked, and your arm is SO STIFF, and SO RIGID, that the harder you try to lower or bend it, the more rigid it becomes. TRY to bend it now and FIND that it just becomes more rigid ...

Allow about three or four seconds ONLY. If you wait too long, you risk either client discomfort, or the possibility of client bending his/her arm.

Now stop trying, and relax all the muscles in your arm. As I count from three down to one, your arm just drops down and you go MUCH deeper into hypnosis.

Gently take client's arm and drop it in his/her lap along with a suggestion to go deeper. Give a suggestion as well for the arm to feel comfortable and relaxed.

WARNING! Do <u>not</u> use this test with anyone who has pain in any part of the wrist, arm or elbow.

Automatic Motion

You should have ascertained during the pre-induction interview which hand is your client's writing hand. (If you don't know, ask now.) Pick up that hand and ask him/her to imagine a piece of chalk between index finger and thumb.

Imagine you are making a series of long, continuous circles on a blackboard.

Start his/her hand rotating as though he/she is actually making circles on a blackboard.

Now continue making those large circles.

Pick up the pace a little, snap your fingers to a FASTER rhythm, suggesting that the hand go faster and faster.

That's good! Now as you continue making these circles, think about your heart. It is beating in response to the needs of your body, and controlled by your subconscious mind. So, also, is your arm being controlled by your subconscious mind... and when I touch your forehead, your arm starts turning in the opposite direction ...

Touch forehead, and say the next word in a paternal way:

REVERSE!

Allow several turns in the opposite direction.

As I touch your forehead again, your arm drops limply to your lap and you go MUCH deeper!

Touch the person's forehead again.

Now just take a deep breath, and relax into a VERY deep, deep, hypnotic sleep. ***

****IMPORTANT NOTES:* If you feel the client was responding to this convincer primarily with the conscious mind, then go right on to another convincer. Also notice that the words "try" and "find" are missing from this test. The reason is because once the subconscious takes control over the circling motion, your client will feel like the subconscious is really controlling the "automatic motion" of the circles – and that helps convince him/her of the trance state. (Use of the analogy of the subconscious controlling involuntary functions increases belief and conviction, enhancing client response.)

Arm Levitation

Pick up client's hand slightly, resting it on your palm

I want you to rest your hand on my palm. Allow me to have the full weight of your arm ... and as I move your arm slowly up

and down, just imagine it getting lighter each time it comes up. Imagine it feels as though it is lighter than air.

Move hand up and down slowly, higher each time. This will actually cause the arm to feel lighter, enhancing the likelihood of hypnotic response.

As soon as your arm floats up off my fingertips, KNOW that you are in hypnosis. Just allow your arm to get lighter each time it comes up. IMAGINE the lightness. FEEL the lightness. And let your subconscious do it for you ... Imagine your arm is beginning to feel as though it's made out of helium balloons and is lighter than air.

Most people will respond before this point. If you sense resistance, you may continue – using more FEELING in your voice in a convincing manner. Then, at your option, you may hold the arm up with one finger and say:

Your arm feels so light that you find it is easy to imagine my finger as a rod of steel which is impossible to push. TRY to push my finger down and FIND that it is impossible. The harder you push, the deeper you go into hypnosis, or the lighter your arm becomes.

Be prepared for the possibility of some pressure on your finger. If client succeeds in pushing your finger down, deepen immediately with Dave Elman floppy arm technique *(described in Chapter 5)* and go right on to another convincer.

Often clients in a somnambulistic state will find their hands floating right off your finger as soon as you tell them to "try" to push. Clients responding to me in this manner will frequently (after awakening from hypnosis) claim to have pushed greatly, or will say that they didn't even try to push because they already knew that they couldn't push down my finger.

To Use Arm Levitation without Touch

Suggest that one arm feels as though it has several dozen helium balloons tied to the wrist, while the other arm feels as though it is made out of lead from the elbow to the fingertips.

> I don't know what's easier for you to imagine ... the lightness or the heaviness ... but the more you imagine either the lightness, or the heaviness, or both, the greater the difference of feeling between your two arms, and the deeper you go into hypnosis. In fact, the slightest movement in your light hand makes you go TEN TIMES DEEPER into hypnosis, until you find your hand feeling so light that it feels as though it could float weightlessly, as you see or feel those helium balloons pulling up on your wrist. Or your heavy arm feels SO HEAVY that it seems as though it would take just too much effort to even try to lift it. So you find it just feels better to simply let it get heavier and heavier ... and the greater the difference of feeling between your two arms, the deeper you go into hypnosis ... (etc.)

What if a Client Fails Two Tests?

If anyone fails two tests, say:

> That's OK ... Just take a deep breath and relax. CHOOSE a deeper state of hypnosis, DESIRE a deeper state of hypnosis, IMAGINE a deeper state of hypnosis, and you WILL go deeper with each suggestion you accept. Now take another deep breath, relaxing completely. Every suggestion you choose to accept takes you deeper and deeper ... or you can simply release, relax, and let go.

At this point, use one or two more deepening techniques, and use several deepening phrases like the ones in the last subsection of Chapter 6 of this book. Then use another hypnotic test. Do not repeat either of the ones just used until there is a response to another, as your client has already proven to himself/herself that the tests can be resisted.

Can Convincers be Used to Measure Hypnotic Depth?

Some scientific researchers of hypnosis use various deepening techniques as well as "challenge" suggestions to measure one's responsiveness and trance depth. With this in mind, various scales have been devised with rigid sets of suggestions. If your motives for learning hypnosis are for scientific advancement, then you may conduct more research to obtain detailed information about the various protocols and hypnotic scales, such as the Stanford Hypnotic Susceptibility Scale, and/or the Harvard scale, etc.

If your motives for learning hypnosis, however, are for helping people change their lives, then perhaps it is wise to decide whether you wish to become an expert in knowledge and scientific research, or whether you wish to devote your time and energies into becoming a <u>*master of the art!*</u> In either case, the *way* you use the techniques is more important than which techniques you use.

Remember: while the scientist uses strict protocols with each subject, the artist adapts to each individual client. One does not have to be an expert scientist in order to estimate whether a client is responding well to suggestions. My own experience proves that measuring exact trance depth with clients is NOT a prerequisite for attaining good results. What's important is that the *belief* of a trance experience contributes to the *expectation* of benefits from the sessions. This will make it easier for the client to *imagine* good results, and become *convinced* that hypnosis works.

Is it a placebo? Perhaps it is. Perhaps all placebos are various forms of self-hypnosis, because of the mind power of the individual. The bottom line, however, is that client-centered hypnosis works. And if skillful use of convincers can strengthen the hypnotic formula, then why not use them?

In Conclusion

Hypnotic tests or "convincers" are important, especially for the client experiencing hypnosis for the first time. In my opinion, for non-medical uses of hypnosis, trance validation for the client is more important than using testing techniques simply to measure the trance state.

There is yet another effective way to help a client become convinced of experiencing the hypnotic state: *the effective use of non-therapeutic post-hypnotic suggestion*. This will be discussed in the next chapter, along with some important guidelines about the structure of suggestions.

Chapter 8

Post-hypnotic Suggestion and Suggestion Structure

One of the most amazing characteristics of hypnosis is the way the subconscious responds to suggestion.

The objectives of this chapter are to provide an overview of the two basic kinds of post-hypnotic suggestion, both non-therapeutic and therapeutic, to show how to use post-hypnotic suggestion as a hypnotic induction, and to discuss suggestion structure itself. Hypnotists use *two styles* of hypnotic suggestions: *direct* suggestion and *indirect* suggestion. Direct suggestion is often paternal, and indirect is usually maternal or permissive; but there can be exceptions both ways.

Before we go any deeper into this chapter, let's put a simple definition on all post-hypnotic suggestion:

> *A post-hypnotic suggestion is any suggestion given to a person while in the state of hypnosis, which is carried out after that person leaves hypnosis.*

Non-therapeutic Post-hypnotic Suggestion

Most therapists consider a non-therapeutic post-hypnotic suggestion to be one that has no direct bearing on therapy, and is *not* necessary for self-improvement.

Outside of a stage hypnotist's use in entertainment, the primary reason for giving most non-therapeutic post-hypnotic suggestions would be as a hypnotic "convincer" to enable the client to validate his/her trance experience. Let's take a look at a common example:

> **After I awaken you from hypnosis, you have an increasing urge to touch your nose one time. If you try to resist, you smile or laugh spontaneously.**

Note the *double bind* (detailed on page 144). The few who try to resist will almost always smile or laugh – and often still end up touching their noses! Also, inclusion of the words "one time" installs a time limit on the suggestion for its automatic removal after only one response (which is considerate).

PLEASE NOTE that you should always be considerate enough to remove any post-hypnotic suggestions that are not beneficial. For example, it would be insensitive to cause someone to scratch his/her nose for the rest of the day! On the other hand, a suggestion to respond alertly to traffic and road situations may benefit the client greatly – yet some hypnotists still consider this to be a non-therapeutic suggestion unless it relates directly to self-improvement. Mr. Tebbetts emphasized on page 252 of the second edition of *Miracles on Demand* the importance of removing all unnatural suggestions:

> *If she should have an accident, such as falling down on a slick floor – although entirely unrelated to the hypnotic session – and the unremoved suggestion had been that her legs were heavy, or stuck to the floor, she could conceivably believe you to be at fault and file suit. It is also possible that a person who hates her job might wish to keep the suggestion that her right arm is too heavy to lift.*

My mentor also emphasized the importance of canceling even those suggestions that a client has rejected, as he believed that when a client leaves your office, he/she should be released from any and all suggestions except those that are beneficial. As previously noted, I agree totally, because a suggestion resisted in the office might cause a response later.

Therapeutic Post-hypnotic Suggestion

Any post-hypnotic suggestion given which is constructive to the therapeutic process and/or directly beneficial for the client is what I consider to be a *therapeutic* post-hypnotic suggestion. For example:

> **Whenever you choose water to satisfy a snack urge, you find yourself satisfied both physically and mentally.**

If hypnosis really caused your client to fall "under your power" then it would be sufficient for you to just describe your client's new desired behavior. But since all hypnosis is really guided self-hypnosis, it's not quite that simple. Even if someone consciously wants to accept a suggestion (with the logical mind), a strong emotional desire to reject a suggestion will result in many of your suggestions going in one ear and out the other. (Remember the "blocks" mentioned at the end of Chapter 2?) This fact is proven by the high backslide rate of 1-session stop-smoking programs. Improper wording (or poor structure) can also neutralize some suggestions; so we will examine that as well in this chapter.

Post-hypnotic Suggestion as a Hypnotic Induction

Many hypnotherapists find it beneficial with certain clients to give post-hypnotic suggestions for instant hypnosis. In my opinion, it is wise to use the combination of *both* a verbal cue and either a visual or kinesthetic trigger, and make it permissive. This provides a measure of safety against hypnotizing someone by accident. For example:

> **Whenever I touch my earlobe (or the back of your hand) and say the words, "DEEP HYPNOSIS," you find that you can immediately go into a deep hypnotic peace.**

Let's examine the above statement. First, it contains the visual or kinesthetic trigger combined with the verbal *trigger for deep hypnosis*. Second, the word "find" enhances the likelihood of results (as explained on page 123). Third, "... you *can* immediately..." is permissive and leaves *choice*, so that your client has the choice to either resist or go ahead and enter hypnosis. (It is usually unwise to hypnotize someone without consent!) Fourth, "... a deep hypnotic peace" suggests that hypnosis provides a peaceful feeling – and in this high-stress society we live in, escape into total peace becomes pleasant and desirable.

Direct and Indirect Suggestion

As previously mentioned, there are two styles of hypnotic suggestions: *direct* suggestion and *indirect* suggestion.

Direct suggestions are like direct requests. Some professionals believe that we give direct suggestions in a paternal way rather than in a permissive or maternal manner; but it is my opinion that any suggestion given as a direct request is a *direct suggestion* even if done in a style that is very maternal. This also includes self-improvement affirmations spoken in the "you are" format rather than "I am" format.

Indirect suggestions are given in a more permissive style, even if done paternally. Metaphors, or stories, often contain indirect suggestions, as the client identifies with parts of the story. One might wonder how or why a story could heal or eliminate pain. *Hypnosis and Hypnotherapy* (Helmut W. A. Karle), contains an interesting example of some Ericksonian hypnosis done over a century before Erickson's birth – by a mother to her child. In 1794, her son developed a tumor that had to be removed surgically. She sat beside him during the surgery and told him a story so interesting that the young boy felt no pain in spite of the fact that no anesthesia was available back then. The surgery was successful. Many years later the boy published the story his mother had told him. The boy was Jacob Grimm. The story was "Snow White."

Much has been written on indirect suggestion as a result of the work of Dr. Milton Erickson, so I will only touch on it here. Charles

Tebbetts primarily used and taught techniques employing direct suggestion. On occasion he used indirect (or permissive) suggestion; but he believed that when people paid their money to go specifically to a *hypnotherapist*, then they would be more prone to respond to direct suggestion than someone seeing either a physician or counselor using hypnosis as an adjunct, when hypnosis was not the original expectation. Although I agree with his reasoning, I use both direct and indirect suggestion, adapting to the client.

Some proponents of indirect suggestion believe that a more permissive style is *always* better. This may be true for some of the people some of the time, but not for all of the people all of the time. It is true that the conscious mind can monitor direct suggestions, but they are easily accepted in the absence of resistance. However, if you have reason to suspect your client might resist even simple suggestions, then an indirect style might be best. On page 75 of *Hypnotic Investigation of Psychodynamic Processes*, Rossi says:

> The reason for the greater effectiveness of indirect suggestion may be formulated as follows: In most trances some consciousness is invariably present in the form of an observer attitude; the subject is in part lost in the experience, but in part the ego is quietly observing what is happening, just as it can in dreams. (p. 75)

If you are a professional desiring to use hypnosis only as an adjunct to your existing practice, and you wish to use primarily indirect suggestion, then I suggest you spend some significant time researching the indirect suggestion techniques mastered by Milton Erickson. Another alternative is to obtain a good script book – or compose your own scripts and get them critiqued by an experienced hypnotherapist or a professional well-versed in Ericksonian hypnotic techniques.

Two excellent books (besides the one just quoted from) for those interested in Dr. Erickson's work are *Experiencing Hypnosis* (Erickson and Rossi), and *Hypnotic Realities* (Erickson and Rossi). Many other books on Ericksonian hypnosis are available.

Charles Tebbetts put some comments concerning indirect suggestion into writing on pages 37–8 (second edition) of *Miracles on Demand* (emphasis mine):

> *An eager beginner gives great reverence to such methods, and they <u>have validity</u>. However, because a method sounds creative, different or profound does not mean it is better than a simpler, tried and true method.*

He told us in class (and wrote in his book) that many of these methods do work; but he believed that they were often an ego trip for the hypnotist. As previously indicated, my own professional views are more modern. I use more indirect suggestions than did my late mentor. During my association with Charles Tebbetts, he frequently expressed the opinion that "profound" techniques satisfied the therapist more than the client, which I believe was the main reason for his using primarily direct suggestions. That being said, one of my former students, well-versed in scientific knowledge and research of hypnosis, is a registered trauma nurse who uses medical applications of hypnosis under medical supervision with patients in hospitals. He uses a considerable amount of direct suggestions, and does so quite effectively.

Early in my hypnotherapy career, I also used primarily direct suggestion; but I've learned to blend both direct and indirect suggestions together, adapting intuitively to my client. As long as the client is happy, that's the bottom line. My recommendation is: *learn and use both.*

On the next page you will find a few examples of both direct and indirect suggestion...

Direct Suggestion	*Indirect Suggestion*
1. As you relax you get so sleepy that you just want to enjoy. Your mind wanders, but your sub-conscious listens to my voice.	1. You can get sleepy or relaxed. You can enjoy, as much as you want to. But you don't need to listen. Just let your mind wander.
2. Now just take a deep breath, and release it. Relax, let go, and just go deeper. You feel a greater sense of deep, hypnotic sleep with each breath that you take.	2. A hiker walking into the woods fills up his lungs with air, noticing that nature is serene and tranquil ... giving him a deeper sense of peace with each breath.
3. Imagine helium balloons tied to your left arm. The more you imagine seeing or feeling the bal-loons, the lighter your arm becomes. Your other arm feels as though it is as heavy as lead, too heavy to even try to lift; and you notice a greater difference of feeling between your two arms.	3. You may notice some-thing interesting happen-ing in one of your arms. Perhaps one of them may feel lighter as if being pulled up by helium bal-loons; or perhaps one of them may feel too heavy to lift. I don't know which feeling is easier for your unconscious to allow you to feel.
4. Close your eyes now, and notice how they just want to stay closed. As your conscious mind drifts and wanders, your subconscious hears and responds to every word I say.	4. It becomes less and less important for your eyes to try to stay open, and your conscious mind can drift or wander while your subconscious hears every word I say, and can cause you to respond.

Constructing Effective Suggestions

In the use of any hypnotic suggestions, Charles Tebbetts believed that both *what* we say and *how* we say it could mean the difference between success and failure. He also felt that, as a general rule, the language should be simple enough for a 12-year old to understand. I concur! He provided some written guidelines for auto-suggestion in Chapter 3 of *Self-Hypnosis and Other Mind-Expanding Techniques*.

I incorporated his philosophy when I wrote the chapters on affirmations in my first self-hypnosis book, *HypnoCise* (self-published in 1986). Affirmations – positive statements of belief – became more popular in the 80s, but all too few seem to know how to structure and use them properly. Since they are like hypnotic suggestions (only in first person format) we should use similar guidelines for maximum effectiveness. My self-hypnosis book *Master the Power of Self-Hypnosis* (Sterling Publishing, 1998) sold over 15,000 copies; and as of the 2010 edition of this book, a newer version is published by Crown House Publishing. Fortunately for me, my first book *predated* Dr. Shad Helmstetter's excellent book, *What to Say When You Talk to Your Self* – which provides credible support to validate many of my own opinions relating to affirmations. I strongly recommend his book to anyone interested in learning more about positive self-talk. (Another book, now out of print, went much deeper into the semantics of hypnotic suggestion: *Psychosemantic Parenthetics* by James F. Russell, Ph.D., who has researched hypnosis for many years.)

Just as poorly constructed affirmations defeat themselves, poorly constructed or misused suggestions could also move client goals further from reach. Wording is vitally important in the structure of suggestions, so let's look closer at some of the basic guidelines for suggestion structure. Some of these guidelines come from Charles Tebbetts, some come from other sources, and some come from my own experience.

Keep the language simple and be specific

When using direct suggestion, state *exactly* what is desired, in simple and specific language. The subconscious is like the "child" in all of us, and children often don't respond well to vague, unclear directions. For example:

With each breath you take, you go deeper and deeper into a deep, hypnotic peace.

A *bad* example would be: *Each time you expand your lung cavity to capacity with air and release it into the atmosphere, you traverse into more of the deeper levels of the more serene somnambulistic trance state, internalizing a greater tranquility.*

What's wrong with this second suggestion?

Some of you may be laughing right now, but I have heard such vague suggestions when I've been on the receiving end of hypnosis! My emotional reaction is much the same as when I'm reading a book written in such pedantic language that even a Ph.D. would have difficulty understanding it.

Even when giving indirect suggestions, it is generally wiser to keep the language simple in most instances.

Keep it positive – suggest the desired result

State the desired result, but *not* what you want avoided.

You find greater satisfaction from the right amounts of those foods which help you reach and maintain your healthiest, ideal weight.

A *bad* example would be: *You don't enjoy eating sweets any more, because you don't want to stay fat.*

What's wrong with this second suggestion?

The language of the subconscious is NOT logic; but rather, it is one of our friendly ingredients of the hypnotic formula, *imagination*. Thus, the suggestion self-destructs by causing the mind to *imagine* sweets and fat. The negative words are usually ignored by the subconscious because of what is known as the *law of reversed effect*.

To illustrate further, say the following statement out loud:

Don't think of a DOG!

Most people will immediately *imagine* seeing a dog, hearing a dog bark, or petting a dog, etc.

A client came to me who went through a quick-fix stop-smoking program. At her request, I listened to the hypnosis tape provided by the facilitator. One suggestion stated emphatically: *"You do not need food as a substitute for smoking."* You guessed it! She was substituting snacks for cigarettes, and had gained 40 pounds in nine months!

A quick way to spot an inadequately trained hypnotist is to listen to the suggestion structure. Even though the best of us can make an occasional slip, some who have taken only a weekend workshop (or less) frequently use negative wording and/or *aversion* suggestions throughout their sessions (or on hypnosis tapes). Somehow they seem to feel that having a smoker wallow around in fantasies of lung cancer and/or crippling strokes will *scare* him/her into quitting – yet this pushes the "rebel" button in some smokers (as reported to me by clients). Worse yet, what happens if they keep on smoking after imagining such horrible diseases?

Charles Tebbetts *RARELY* gave aversion suggestions.

What is expected tends to be realized

This is called: *the law of expectancy.*

One basic natural law is that we tend to get whatever we believe or expect at a subconscious level. This applies to hypnotic suggestion just as in affirmations. When we construct hypnotic suggestions in a way that feeds into the *expectation* of our clients, we have another vital ingredient of the hypnotic formula working – especially after several previous hypnotic responses ...

Just as you found your arm dropping when you imagined the bucket, you can also find your arm getting lighter now by imagining helium balloons.

Artful use of *compounding suggestions* can also increase the expectation and likelihood of acceptance of therapeutic post-hypnotic suggestions. Each suggestion responded to *during* the hypnotic state increases the client's expectation of continued automatic responses, as in the following examples of direct suggestion and indirect suggestion ...

It's natural for your body to have water ... so whenever you choose water to satisfy snack urges, you find it becomes totally satisfying, because you love your power of choice.

Is it necessary for you to find those urges diminishing immediately? You may have been surprised when your arm felt lighter. Won't you also be surprised when you wake up some morning and find yourself feeling like a non-smoker?

Emphasize and emotionalize (say it with FEELING)

Charles Tebbetts used to say, "Exaggerate and emotionalize." He taught that we should use words such as *wonderful, beautiful, great, joyous, tremendous*, etc., and say them with *feeling*. In other words, go with the flow, and flow with it. When I facilitated student sessions at Charlie's hypnotism school, others seemed to respond faster when I followed his advice and spoke with feeling – much more than when I used a monotone voice.

How do you give suggestions with *feeling?*

First, you can *emphasize* certain words. Second, and far more critical, you should *project yourself into the importance* of the suggestions. Allow yourself to *feel* the art *intuitively*. For example, tell your client that it *feels good* to go into deep hypnosis, etc. Also, learn enough techniques so well that they just become like second nature to you – so that you can literally go into a light state of self-hypnosis yourself when you work with someone.

My voice coach used to tell me to *feel* the music I was singing. This was difficult until I learned the piece of music and could sing it from my "right brain" instead of from my conscious mind. There were just too many musical concerns for me to think about until the music flowed so easily that I could literally go into *alpha* and let my *feelings go with the flow*. Also, it helped me to project into the message, or the meaning of the music. When I facilitate hypnosis, I also project into the meaning and impact of what I say. When suggesting success, I imagine my client being successful!

There can be no pretense on this issue if you are using hypnosis in an analytical way purely from a technical frame of reference. Strict scientific protocol may inhibit your ability to feel an art, especially if you are working totally from the "left brain." You may miss some important opportunities to adapt wisely to your client if you close down your intuition.

If it is absolutely essential for you to be precise, then choose (or write) your script ahead of time and stick to it. Become familiar enough with its content so that you can still emphasize certain words and speak with feeling.

Many hypnosis professionals use prepared scripts. There are literally thousands of scripts available, and numerous script books. Before using any of them, read carefully prior to use and be prepared to edit as necessary according to the guidelines of effective suggestion. As you edit, remember the most important concept: *imagination is the language of the subconscious*. What will the client *imagine* as a result of your script? If you wish to see some sample scripts that include indirect suggestion and metaphors, Paul Durbin has some posted at: www.durbinhypnosis.com/script/

htm. Again, be sure to edit any script before use, even one that you write yourself.

Should we use present tense?

For years I avoided using the word "will" altogether in giving suggestions – as is apparent to anyone who has read my older self-hypnosis book. However, experience demonstrates that we may use the word "will" when linked to a *specified time, event,* or *trigger* (action), and still have a good likelihood of increasing the subconscious response.

Linking the desired result to an *undefined* future time or place, however, may not be as productive. By making the statement, *"Tomorrow you will control your eating habits,"* you give the subconscious permission to wait until tomorrow; and we all know that tomorrow never comes!

If you give the subconscious an escape hatch, it usually finds a way to use it – so use caution with future tense. This is especially important when using direct suggestions. If there is a need for future tense (such as with a heavily overweight client), use *progressive* tense such as either: *Every day your body is getting closer to reaching and maintaining its ideal weight;* OR: *You are becoming more like your ideal self with each passing day.*

Should you be active or passive?

When using autosuggestion, it is better to use active statements (or affirmations) rather than passive ones. I *can* sing. Does that tell you that I actually do sing? I can also cook – when I get around to it. (God bless microwaves!)

With hypnotic suggestion, however, there are times when it can be both appropriate and desirable to be passive and/or permissive. "Can" is a passive and/or permissive word, and has a valid place in any type of suggestion you give when the client needs to maintain choice and/or enjoy an increased ability to respond. (Refer to the subsection "Post-hypnotic Suggestion as a Hypnotic Induction" in this chapter for an example of how to use the word "can" for choice.)

Direct suggestions *actively* suggest the desired result:

Close your eyes, take a deep breath, and relax.

An indirect suggestion passively or *permissively* suggests the desired result as an ability or a choice:

When you are ready, you <u>can</u> allow your eyes to close, and notice how easy it is to take a deep breath and relax.

Just as with hypnotic suggestions for response *during* hypnosis, there are two schools of thought on whether a therapeutic post-hypnotic suggestion should be active (direct) or passive (indirect). I am now neutral on this, as I believe in adapting to each individual client. If desired, you could lessen the likelihood of resistance by *preceding* your induction with a permissive suggestion or question such as:

Would you like to extend the foot rest on the recliner so that you can enjoy a deeper state of hypnosis?

Note by the above example that *questions* may serve as *indirect suggestions!* You may wish to consider using some very powerful permissive suggestions, such as a double bind ...

The EITHER/OR choice, or the double bind

This combines the best of salesmanship with hypnosis. Milton Erickson is credited with frequent use of double binds, but properly trained salespeople know how to reduce the possibility of getting a "no" by saying, "In your price range, I can give you *either* the brown *or* the blue one. Which do you prefer?" This same principle applies in hypnosis, as the hypnotic artist *sells* suggestions to the subconscious ...

You may feel your arm getting lighter while you go deeper into hypnosis, or you may prefer to let it feel very heavy as you drift down into a deep trance.

Some people consider this a form of *indirect* suggestion because it involves choice; but the double bind contains two direct suggestions with the "either/or" choice. So which is it? You decide. Perhaps we should call it direct suggestion given in a permissive way – or *permissive direct suggestion*. In either case, the double bind is a powerful suggestion. In my opinion, results are more important than labels!

Avoid words with double meanings

The subconscious knows no jokes, so we should say *exactly* what we desire – avoiding slang expressions or words with double meanings. Consider a seemingly acceptable suggestion: *"Your good eating habits help you lose excess weight."*

Can you see the subtle subconscious escape hatch here? We were programmed as children to try to *find* what we lose! Yet many people keep losing weight, only to find it again year after year. We can reduce, discard, release, throw away, give away, take off, get rid of, eliminate, or donate excess pounds; but if we think we lost weight, our subconscious will go looking for it again. A better way of stating this is:

Your good eating habits enable you to reduce easily.

Furthermore, unexpected client resistance after initial success could result from a word that has a negative meaning from your client's viewpoint even though that word might be generally positive. For example, one of my own clients kept popping right out of hypnosis every time I started deepening techniques. After four sessions where I just consulted her on the use of self-hypnotic suggestions, she realized that she had a phobia regarding the word "deeper" because of falling into a well when she was a small child. When I used the words "more mellow" instead, she went into somnambulism.

Also, "pride" is a negative word to some people because of religious training – but *very positive* to other people!

Be considerate and ethical

Some hypnotists seem to think that it's "cute" to give bizarre post-hypnotic suggestions. In one demonstration, a hypnotist put a pencil eraser on the hand of a volunteer and told him it was a burning cigarette – and a painful blister formed. Even though the hypnotist boasted a *Ph.D.* behind his name, this suggestion, in my opinion, served neither the volunteer nor the audience. It was an embarrassment to the hypnotherapy profession, and created fear with observers. Most professional hypnosis associations have ethical codes prohibiting such insensitive suggestions.

Always give only those suggestions you would be willing to respond to if your roles were reversed.

This is a good lead-in to the next chapter.

Chapter 9

Ethics and Potential Dangers

Hypnotic ethics could be summarized in one statement: *do for the client what you would want done if your roles were reversed.*

If every hypnotist diligently applied the golden rule to all uses of hypnosis, I could end the chapter right here and make it one of the shortest chapters ever written for a book. Unfortunately, human nature makes it too easy to get sidetracked; consequently, an entire book could be written on this subject alone – so I suggest that you keep on reading.

We often hear that hypnosis is not dangerous. If every hypnotist always gave only ethical suggestions, no discussion of dangers would be necessary; but since that's not the case, we must also consider some of the real and imagined dangers of hypnosis resulting from the unwise use of suggestions.

What Constitutes Ethics?

All valid professional hypnosis associations have codes of ethics that their memberships must agree to abide by. While various ethical codes may have slight variations from one another, they contain the same basic professional objectives: do what is good for the client, maintain client confidentiality, avoid harmful techniques, etc., and use other common-sense guidelines. While I may not agree with all the policies of the National Guild of Hypnotists, their code of ethics published in the 1990s shines as an example of how a typical client-centered code of ethics should be written; so I discuss it in my hypnotherapy class. (Other associations also have similar ethical codes.)

The N.G.H. Code of Ethics and Standards

I. General Principles:
A. *The physical and mental well-being of each client shall always be a prime consideration.*
   Here again is the golden rule of hypnosis: do for the client what you would want done if the roles were reversed.

B. *The rights and desires of the client shall always be respected.*
   Same comment as above.

C. *Members shall avoid any conduct which could be construed as moral impropriety or sexual misconduct with a client.*
   This could be very costly if you end up in a court of law.

D. *Members shall use hypnosis strictly within the limits of their training and competence.*
   Any hypnotherapist not doing this could be gambling with his/her career.

E. *Members shall be honest and ethical in their advertising and business dealings.*
   A false ad may get a quick buck, but ultimately you will pay for it. When hypnotherapy is misrepresented, it reflects poorly on the profession in the eyes of the general public, and hurts our profession in the eyes of the general public.

F. *Hypnosis shall be employed in accordance with established laws and regulations.*
   Let's do what we can to keep hypnosis legal!

G. *Members shall be aware of their limitations and always avoid infringement on other professions.*
   It would be inconsiderate of your client for you to refrain from referring him/her elsewhere when appropriate. My own experience shows that clients respect the integrity of staying within one's qualifications.

H. *Professional behavior and respect should be extended to all fellow hypnotists.*
We are in a people-helping profession. Let's be more helpful to each other as well.

II. *Practice of Hypnosis:*
A. *Members shall establish and maintain proper records necessary to a professional practice.*
Check with state, city and county governments for appropriate business licenses and/or any record-keeping requirements. Also, be sure to keep client records confidential and locked. If your office is ever vandalized (as mine was), then obtain a copy of the police report in order to document when and why any records were compromised.

B. *Members shall use hypnosis with clients to motivate them to eliminate negative or unwanted habits, facilitate the learning process, improve memory and concentration, develop self-confidence, eliminate stage fright, improve athletic abilities, and for other social, educational and cultural endeavors of a <u>non-medical</u> nature, unless to do otherwise is within the limits of their training and competence (emphasis mine).*
I always emphasize a *non-medical* nature to my students. Pain is a warning that something is wrong with the body, and the source of the pain needs to be diagnosed by someone who is competent and licensed to do so.

The N.G.H. code also specifies the following: avoid harmful inductions; demonstrate hypnosis in a tasteful way; avoid shocking and/or sudden awakenings; remove unnecessary suggestions; employ positive (rather than negative) post-hypnotic suggestions; avoid age-regression unless trained in this area; avoid forensic hypnosis unless adequately trained in that field of study; avoid suggestions for hallucinations which could be frightening, shocking, obscene, sexually suggestive, degrading or humiliating.

In addition, the code defines other professional behavior. There is nothing in the N.G.H. code of ethics that any professional using hypnosis shouldn't already be doing or avoiding, if he or she is sincerely serving the client; but *one other ethical issue* is of such importance that it requires an entire chapter section.

"Hypnotic Seal"

The N.G.H. Code of Ethics and Standards *prohibits giving suggestions to a client blocking the induction of hypnosis by another*, as this infringes on the rights of that client (II-*H*-2); yet, as incredible as it seems, certain experts in the scientific community have actually used and advocated this unethical practice! The alleged motive is "protection" from a lay hypnotist; but such a block disempowers the recipient. Myron Teitelbaum calls it the *hypnotic seal*, and he discussed it in detail in *Hypnosis Induction Technics.* (pp. 104–110).

Some years ago a student in my class was unable to respond to any hypnotic techniques in spite of her desire to do so. We soon realized that she had been given a seal. Breaking the seal took several steps.

First, I showed her a copy of my membership certificate in a professional hypnosis association, proving to her subconscious that I was trained in the art of hypnosis. Then I used suggestibility tests to help her understand the role of imagination in the hypnotic process. After reminding her that all hypnosis is guided self-hypnosis, and that she would be actually *hypnotizing herself* by using my words as a guide, she could now allow herself to enter hypnosis.

Once hypnotized, she easily accepted my suggestions to respond to any other professional hypnotherapist or student of hypnosis whenever *she chose* to be hypnotized. I broke the seal by *giving her the power of choice.*

If you strongly believe that you might have valid reason to put such a seal on a patient or client (to inhibit unwanted hypnosis), give him/her a simple trance-prevention trigger to use IF and when *he or she chooses*. This is far better than infringing on that person's personal freedom of choice.

Ethics Legislated in Washington State

Hypnotherapists in Washington State are legally required to follow the ethical *Uniform Disciplinary Code*. I believe that other states could benefit from emulating this example.

This state produced a flier, written in easy language, suitable for distribution to a client. It discusses client and counselor responsibilities and rights. It encourages you and your counselor or hypnotherapist to discuss the type of counseling expected; the methods or techniques that might be used; the therapist's education, training and experience; and the cost of counseling sessions.

The hypnotherapist or counselor must provide written information that explains these topics, allowing the client to read the information and sign a statement acknowledging same. Additionally, the state-approved flier must either be given to the client or posted where the client can easily read it.

The definition of professional conduct is then spelled out by Washington State for the new client. The flier informs the client about what kind of professional conduct is prohibited...

Abuse of a client or sexual contact with a client.

Incompetence, negligence or malpractice that harms a client or creates an unreasonable risk of harm to a client.

Willful betrayal of a practitioner-client privilege as recognized by law.

The commission of any act involving moral turpitude, dishonesty or corruption relating to the practice of counseling or hypnotherapy. The act does not have to be a crime in order to be a violation of the law regulating counselors and hypnotherapists.

Practicing counseling or hypnotherapy while suffering from a contagious or infectious disease in a way that would pose a serious risk to public health.

Aiding a client to obtain an abortion through illegal means.

Possession, use or distribution of drugs except for a legitimate purpose, addiction to drugs or violation of any drug law.

Habitual use of or impairment from the use of alcohol.

Misrepresentation or fraud in any aspect of the conduct of the profession.

Advertising that is false, fraudulent or misleading.

Offering to treat clients by a secret method, procedure or treatment.

Although many hypnotherapists initially feared the new legislation, it has proven beneficial for both the public and the hypnotherapy profession since 1988.

The law requires both basic ethics as well as full disclosure to clients as to the hypnotherapist's training, education, experience, professional associations, etc. This legislation also discourages the charlatans from making hyped-up false claims about hypnosis by prohibiting false advertising.

For some reason, however, this has not yet stopped all of the "hotel hoppers" from claiming 97 percent success rates in ads for their aversion stop-smoking programs. Since most people don't seem to read the fine print in the ads, many of them – who want something quick, cheap and "guaranteed" – go to such programs, only to end up believing that hypnosis is a scam because they still want a cigarette.

Can you make a quick buck in hypnosis if you know how to market with such misleading ads? ...yes, unless you get into legal trouble for false advertising. Are you doing the public and the hypnotherapy profession a favor?

My response is: Please refer your participants to *local hypnotherapists* for the badly-needed follow-up sessions! Let's create a multi-win.

There are additional prohibited actions spelled out in Washington beyond what I've quoted here; but I will comment on only one more prohibited act:

> *Promotion for personal gain of any drug, device, treatment, procedure or service that is unnecessary or has no acceptable benefit to the client.*

Some network marketing organizations entice health care professionals to sell health food or supplements to clients and patients. If you attempt to market products to your clients for personal gain, it may be in your best interests to consult with an attorney. Some hypnotherapy clients might perceive it as a breach of professionalism to be told to buy "Nutri-Off" or "Macro-Eat", etc., etc. Also, the sale of tablets to allegedly reduce withdrawals from nicotine could be construed as prescribing.

In Washington State, you could get into deep trouble (and may be in violation of the Uniform Disciplinary Code) because of improper sales of products in your office. If you are in network marketing, you may offer hypnotherapy to your customers and your down line, but it is a professional risk to try to push such products onto your hypnosis clients. (Hypnosis tapes, CDs and books are OK to sell or give to clients.)

Is Hypnosis Dangerous?

Many professional hypnotherapists agree with the opinion held by Charles Tebbetts, that hypnosis of and by itself is not dangerous. My mentor often stated that not one documented case of someone being harmed by hypnosis had ever been presented to him. At the same time, he recognized the fact that the misuse of suggestion to remove pain could be detrimental to a client (*Miracles on Demand*, p. 43). For example, masking headache pain just because a client wanted relief could prevent early detection of a brain tumor; so Mr. Tebbetts taught his students to always have a written medical consent from the client's examining physician before using any medical applications of hypnosis.

John C. Hughes, in *The Induction of Conviction*, concurred by saying:

> *Hypnosis in and of itself is not at all dangerous. The only possible danger is in the misuse of suggestion. The responsible and adequately trained hypnotherapist, through judicious use of appropriate suggestion, will avoid any difficulty in his or her use of hypnosis. So are there people using hypnosis without adequate training? The answer is unfortunately in the affirmative; however, even people with advanced degrees often engage in hypnosis without having had adequate training! And the advanced degree is not a substitute for training in the art of hypnosis.*

This brings up a very controversial question for both real and imagined dangers of hypnosis...

Just What Constitutes Adequate Training?

There are many thousands of competently trained hypnotherapists helping people make profound changes in their lives through the skilled use of appropriate suggestion. Many who have only B.A. degrees (or even less) have invested in specialized vocational training in the use of hypnotism – recognized and credentialed by one or several professional hypnosis associations. Yet as discussed earlier in my book, there are some hypnotherapists with graduate degrees in psychology or medicine who complain that only people with advanced degrees should practice hypnotherapy because of the "dangers" of hypnosis. Charles Francis, M.A., A.C.H., considers this position totally unwarranted, as stated on page 79 of his book, *Counseling Hypnotherapy: The Synergism of Psychotherapy and Hypnotherapy*...

> *Many psychologists and physicians who use hypnosis are minimally trained in that field. Studies of hypnosis are not usually requirements of graduate or medical degree programs. Hypnotherapy has proved itself and grown in value and recognition to the point where it can and should stand on its own feet. But competency should be required and verified by training organizations.*

As of the first revision of this book, most professional hypnosis associations agreed upon an industry standard of a minimum of *100 hours of hypnosis education + practice hours + annual ongoing education*. While I feel the standard may someday be higher, I support this major step forward.

Even now, some hypnotherapy instructors invest time and effort in their training programs by submitting their curriculum to one or more of the various hypnosis organizations for approval or certification. (Over the years, I have personally submitted my course curriculum to several different hypnotherapy associations, including the International Medical and Dental Hypnotherapy Association, and a state association – the Washington Hypnosis Association. Tacoma Community College also had to approve the course.)

Such professional approval from any credible organization is usually dependent on both the number of hours the hypnotherapy instructor includes in the training program as well as the content of material taught.

There are many self-appointed hypnosis instructors, however, who take short cuts and create their own self-certifying "associations" rather than investing the necessary time and effort to submit a course curriculum to a recognized hypnosis association for approval. Worse, some people claim to "train and certify" after only a crash course of just one or two weekends, and then tell participants to set up practice. One large hypnosis association engaged in this policy throughout the 1980s and 1990s.

People who go through such programs are taking their chances on the quality of training. Even when sophisticated academic and scientific information is included in such courses, there is *no substitute for practice* to master an art. Anyone not previously trained in hypnosis should consider a weekend course as *only an introduction* to the hypnotherapy profession.

In 1991 an internist told me that he had gone to a weekend hypnosis training program to become a "Certified Medical Hypnotherapist." He said this program was open only to physicians and people with other doctoral degrees. He stated that a few interesting medical applications of hypnosis were presented, but added that his degree in medicine did not substitute for the lack of thorough training in the art of hypnosis.

I respect those who have earned advanced degrees; but I take exception to those who put the label of "lay hypnotist" on a full-time professional who is competently trained and dedicated to the hypnotherapy profession. There are claims of "lay hypnotists" harming people. Well, how many people die on operating tables? ...and how many patients spend many years in psychotherapy, with little or no improvement?

Sarcasm aside, I will not attempt to defend any misuse of hypnosis. However, some of the most inconsiderate uses (or abuses) of hypnosis that others have brought to my attention have surprisingly been made by people with either "M.D." or "Ph.D." behind their names. That surprises some people.

Do Advanced Degrees Ensure Wise Use of Hypnosis?

A smoker who saw me in 1987 said that he had seen a physician for hypnosis a year earlier (rather than a hypnotherapist) because his insurance company only covered hypnosis when performed by a licensed physician. My client said that he had a vivid memory of that physician suggesting "toxic pollutants" poisoning his lungs, creating cancerous tissue – and he was told to visualize this while he was in a state of hypnosis! He continued smoking in spite of the aversion suggestions, but did not return to this doctor. By the time he saw me, he complained of frequent pain in his lungs. I advised him to consult a licensed physician for the pain in his lungs, but I did accept him as a client for smoking cessation. After going a full month without smoking, he told me that my hypnosis program saved his former doctor from a malpractice suit.

Another case of insensitive suggestion was given by a psychiatrist who told his patient that she would get nauseous every time she tasted or smelled pizza. Since she was desperate to overcome her pizza addiction at the time, her subconscious bought the suggestion. Unfortunately, both her husband and teenager loved to have pizza delivered several times weekly, which resulted in her leaving the room and losing whatever was in her stomach. This went on for over a year before she finally got enough courage to see a hypnotherapist and have the suggestion reversed. I asked her why she didn't go back to her psychiatrist right after she realized the inconvenience, and her response was, "I didn't trust him anymore." (Would you?)

Another unwise use of hypnosis was reported to me by an experienced hypnotherapist. A psychologist hypnotized one of her clients for a fear of swimming, and then gave him a "shock" suggestion to imagine being sucked into a giant whirlpool at sea. The next evening, after finishing his bath, he looked at the small whirlpool caused by the water going down the drain, and went into a psychotic episode.

In yet another case, a woman previously abused by several male authority figures saw a Ph.D. who told her – while she was hypnotized – that she was rebellious, and he ordered her to obey his suggestions! The female therapist who discussed this case with me informed me that the woman was ruined for seeing male therapists after this incident.

I've already discussed the insensitive example of another Ph.D. creating a painful blister (see last subsection of Chapter 8). Also, let's consider the "hypnotic seal" discussed earlier in this chapter and pose a serious question: how many people are running around thinking that they cannot be hypnotized because they have been given a seal by some inconsiderate hypnotist?

Now let's examine what some experts in the scientific community consider to be potential dangers of hypnosis. I also discuss some of this same information in the official FAQ (Frequently Asked Questions) of the "alt.hypnosis" newsgroup on the internet. The official FAQ is stored on my website: http://www.royhunter. com/hypnofaq.htm.

Potential of mental illness

The risk of positive suggestion creating a mental illness is, in my opinion, almost non-existent for the clients of any hypnotherapist <u>using common sense</u> and being considerate of the client. However, using bizarre programmed imagery in a negative way is a question of ethics and/or lack of training in hypnotherapy. The Ph.D. who used negative suggestion in the whirlpool incident certainly had training in psychology, but apparently little or no training in hypnotherapy. Also, did the psychiatrist who gave his patient the aversion suggestion about pizza use either common sense or suggestions that were considerate? Had he gone through a comprehensive *professional hypnotherapy* training program, maybe he would have realized that such insensitive aversion suggestions would cause a great inconvenience to his patient.

Being considerate of clients – as well as using common sense with suggestions – should eliminate this as a concern for the adequately trained hypnotherapist, whether or not the hypnotherapist has an advanced degree.

Also bear in mind that those who are told in advance of hypnotherapy that *all hypnosis is really guided self-hypnosis* will be much more likely to reject any suggestions they don't want, because that belief becomes more empowering. This may not be as true, however, for someone who enters hypnosis with the erroneous belief that a medical authority is in control of his/her mind during the hypnotic state. People *respond according to their beliefs*; and through *ignorance* a person could be duped into giving away more control than necessary – thus giving the unethical hypnotist virtual control over the subject who subjects himself to that erroneous belief.

Causing hypnotic regression

A hypnotic regression is like a memory "flashback" in time. All of us can experience this when watching a motion picture that reminds us of a childhood memory. Some years back, the movie *Platoon* caused many Vietnam veterans to have vivid regressions, along with emotional feelings, called abreactions. (Perhaps every motion picture theater should have an attending psychologist present whenever a movie is shown in case people have abreactions.)

First of all, let's consider the fact that a trained hypnotherapist might, in some cases, choose to hypnotize a client with a hypnotic regression, this being *one of the objectives* to achieving therapeutic results! This is perfectly acceptable if the hypnotherapist is trained in the effective handling of client abreactions, understands the risk of false memory syndrome, AND works within his/her areas of competency.

The hypnotist who is not trained in regression therapy, however, is well advised to avoid deliberate use of hypnotic suggestion to cause a regression. Furthermore, hypnotic regressions are prohibited in some codes of ethics unless one has received training in regression therapy. Why is this so? The primary reason is the risk of false memories ...

If a hypnotist improperly leads the client, fantasies could become mixed with memories – and a father's innocent hug could be perceived as a sexual molestation. If you cause this, you'd better have malpractice insurance! Also, you'd better know how to properly facilitate a client's abreactions before you attempt hypnotic regressions – otherwise your client could leave your office emotionally upset – or *worse.*

Many hypnotists do NOT intentionally initiate hypnotic regressions ... but what about the rare *accidental* regressions where that was not the original intent? If this happens to a hypnotist untrained in regression therapy, the client should be kept in hypnosis and taken (in the imagination) to a safe or peaceful place. Suggestions of general well-being can then be given, along with suggestions to choose *wisely* when and how to deal with the issues – at the most appropriate time and place. (The peaceful place is covered in Chapter 10.)

Making a disorder worse by symptom removal

Any competent hypnotherapy instructor emphasizes to his or her students the importance of requiring a written referral from an examining physician before ever using hypnosis to reduce pain or to attempt to remove physical symptoms. The exception (for those who are not licensed to practice medicine) is if the examining physician is physically present and/or is supervising the hypnotic process. Since pain is a warning that something is wrong with the body, the cause must be discovered by someone who is licensed to diagnose.

Once the client brings the medical referral, hypnotherapy may help considerably.

A woman suffering from arthritis as well as chronic back pain from an auto accident came to me for help. She brought a written referral from her physician to learn self-hypnosis for managing her pain. After four sessions, she was able to reduce her pain in a dramatic way; but with the seriousness of her back injury, her own mind kept just enough of her pain active to prevent further injury. The cost of her pain medication reduced from $120 down to about $50 monthly, and both she and her doctor were happy.

I also know a certified hypnotherapist with a Ph.D. who specializes in hypnotherapy for helping people who suffer from catastrophic illness, provided they bring the appropriate referrals from their examining physicians. Also, as mentioned earlier in this book, Paul Durbin, Ph.D., actually spent years working with patients inside hospitals in the South, and eventually become the Director of Clinical Hypnotherapy at the Methodist Hospital in New Orleans. (He is both a personal friend and a man of high integrity, as well as a published author.)

I believe there is a virtually untapped market with the hundreds of thousands of people suffering from major disease; but it is very important to work cooperatively with the medical community in this area rather than to trying to bypass it.

Hopefully we can build a better bridge between traditional medicine and hypnotherapy. Meanwhile, I warn all of my students to avoid crossing the "invisible line" between appropriate hypnotherapy and unlicensed practice of medicine. The medical use of hypnosis (by someone not medically licensed) is a violation of ethical codes of most professional hypnosis associations, and could also result in a client getting worse (and/or potential legal complications). However, whenever a medical application of hypnosis IS appropriate, a competently trained hypnotherapist does not just remove symptoms. Instead, he/she will usually first find out whether there is a subconscious cause that must be released, in order to reduce the possibility of the symptom returning. This hypnotic process is discussed in my advanced text, *The Art of Hypnotherapy* (also available from Crown House Publishing).

Criminal activity

No ethical hypnotherapist would even consider trying to use hypnosis to induce criminal or anti-social behavior, or trying to trick someone into doing such. (Someone can be tricked whether or not in trance.) Research seems to indicate that a person refuses obvious suggestions to break the law *unless* he/she is already inclined to do so. Military use may appear otherwise, but only because the soldier has already decided to follow orders to kill for his country if necessary.

Forensic hypnosis

If you plan on using forensic hypnosis, perhaps you should read *Trance on Trial* (Scheflin and Shapiro) and then decide whether you wish to seek additional training in that field first. Unless you have a background in law or law enforcement, be sure the training you receive is both specialized and adequate. Even with all my years of experience in hypnotherapy, I still avoid the use of forensic hypnosis. This is a specialized area that requires specialized training!

Excessive dependence or danger of prolonged treatment

The dependence issue should not be a concern with any client of a hypnotherapist who seeks to help a client become *self-empowered*. Although I have no knowledge of alleged "mind control" experiments that some people claim are taking place, I oppose using hypnosis for disempowerment. Client-centered techniques are designed to help clients use the *power of their own minds* to change, with the hypnotherapist acting merely as the guide or facilitator.

Hypnosis is a very important part of my own success in life. Am I dependent on it? Well, my life would not be the same without it! I frequently use self-hypnosis, which is like a muscle. If I move a chair, I can easily lift it – but when I move a couch, it's easier if someone on the other end is helping me lift it. So when I seem stuck in an obstacle preventing me from reaching a goal, I quickly swallow my pride and seek hypnotherapy from another professional!

When we go to school, we are educated on how to use our left brains with knowledge, intelligence, and hopefully some wisdom as well; but few of us are ever taught how to use our right brains in a positive manner. Self-empowering hypnosis can help a client reach a greater potential, especially if the secrets of self-hypnosis are wisely shared.

Highly motivated people often use self-hypnosis without even knowing that they are doing so. Also, much has been written on visualization for healing and self-help; and even the scientific community realizes the power of using the right brain. Two examples are *Healing Visualizations: Creating Healing Through Imagery* (Gerald Epstein, M.D.), and *Love, Medicine, & Miracles* (Bernie Siegel, M.D.). Another outstanding book on visualization is *Creative Visualization* by Shakti Gawain, written more as a "how to" book with some philosophical concepts than as an academic treatise.

Now let's discuss the danger of using hypnosis to prolong treatment. Any hypnotherapist working from a center of love wouldn't dream of using hypnosis to prolong treatment; however, some years back I was informed of a credentialed psychotherapist who gave her clients hypnotic suggestions to keep on returning weekly for over a year. One of her clients told me personally that the only risk of the enjoyable long series of sessions was to her own pocketbook; however, it is my opinion that her therapist's motives could have been called into question. While I wish this was an isolated case, the day after Rabin was assassinated, a Seattle newspaper ran a front-page article about a licensed mental health counselor using hypnosis who kept a woman in session 147 times. I wonder where he got his hypnosis training.

Sexual fantasies

Not only would it be unwise to give sexually suggestive suggestions to any client, it is also a violation of the Uniform Disciplinary Code as well as ethical codes of any credible hypnosis association.

It's apparently common, however, for some women to fantasize affairs with doctors. This opinion came from some of the women I dated when I was single. They knew, because they often engaged in such fantasies and told me so. (I have not taken a poll of my clients to ask them this same question concerning hypnotherapists; nor do I intend to do so.)

Can a man or a woman in hypnosis have sexual fantasies? When you consider that many people don't even need to be in hypnosis to indulge in sexual fantasies, the answer should be obvious. Common sense alone should tell the prudent person to avoid giving any suggestions which could possibly be perceived by a client as sexually suggestive.

Be Non-Judgmental of Your Clients

Charles Tebbetts advised us to work with clients without showing any prejudice or criticism, so that clients feel free of being judged or criticized. He felt that if any one of us were born into the body of a client and had the same experiences, we would react in the same ways – and therefore we should always put ourselves into the shoes of our clients. Furthermore, if our clients feel that we are criticizing them for their problems, rapport is difficult at best. Worse, we could damage the client's self-esteem.

We must also respect the beliefs of our clients. A woman complained to me because another hypnotherapist criticized her for requesting a "past life" regression.

If a client believes that his or her problem originated in a former lifetime, then you should either work within the framework of your client's beliefs or *refer* him/her to someone who will! Refusing in a critical manner on the grounds that it is neither "scientific" nor Christian may be very offensive if you fail to refer.

If a prospective client has opinions and ideas that inhibit your ability to stay objective, other therapists may be more comfortable – and effective – in territory where skeptics fear to tread. Clients do not come to have their religious beliefs criticized because of your conflicting spiritual, religious, scientific or philosophical ideas.

Unless you are an ordained minister and someone comes to you for spiritual counseling, be *extremely careful* what you say about religion and/or "new age" ideas, or you may be treading on very thin ice! Whether or not you believe in past life therapy, your client deserves either help or a referral – but NOT criticism.

Assumptions can also be risky ...

Several clients have complained to me over the years because of another hypnotherapist trying to convince them that their problems originated in another life. In my opinion it is a breach of ethics to intentionally attempt a "past life" regression with a client who has not specifically requested it.

Assuming that someone believes in Christ can also be a mistake. Several years ago I assumed that a client was a Christian when she talked about "praying to God" for help with her problem during the pre-talk. She had difficulty releasing the cause; so I unwisely suggested that she release her fear into the "Christ light" – and this would give her faith to increase her confidence.

She brought herself immediately up out of deep trance, saying, *"I'm Jewish, and I resent your using the name of Christ in this session!"*

Even though she accepted my apology, rapport was broken, and she would not go back into hypnosis. Worse, she failed to refer any of her employees to me as previously promised. I unknowingly criticized her beliefs by calling on Christ, and it cost me several thousand dollars of lost referral business.

This is a "learning experience" that I share with my own students so that they do not have to reinvent the wheel.

In Conclusion

The degree of education does not guarantee ethical use of hypnosis; *motives and personal integrity* influence ethics. Is the hypnotherapist coming from a love center? Will the therapist have the common sense to stay within his or her qualifications?

My advice to the new hypnosis student is that you wait until you have training in a technique before you attempt to use it. This is especially true with regressions – as mentioned before – because of the risk of false memories. Regressions require the therapist to understand the difference between guiding and leading, AND to know how to competently deal with abreactions. Sometimes students of the art of hypnosis want to jump ahead; but in the long run, I believe that you will find your patience is worth the end result.

Please do not short-cut your training. Pay your dues. Master some basic techniques of the art of hypnosis before practicing hypnotherapy. Both you and your clients will benefit from this investment of your time!

Chapter 10

Self-hypnosis for Stress Coping

One of the more enjoyable evenings I experienced at The Charles Tebbetts Hypnotism Training Institute was the class on self-hypnosis training.

Mr. Tebbetts spent part of the evening reviewing some of the same material from his first book, *Self-Hypnosis and Other Mind-Expanding Techniques*. Originally self-published, Westwood Publishing took over the first edition and sold several hundred thousand copies. After disputes over the copyright, it has been published both in its original form and in a revised version, both by Mr. Tebbetts and by others several times since its original printing. As of the writing of this book, I believe it is still available through Westwood Publishing. I highly recommend it to my own students, as well as to all professional hypnotherapists.

At Edmonds, my mentor first discussed the five methods of subconscious programming – which I have incorporated into my "benefits approach" to motivation, and teach in Part II of *Diversified Client-Centered Hypnosis*. (I also discuss these briefly in the next chapter, which preserves certain concepts of the mind that Mr. Tebbetts felt that all hypnosis students need to understand.)

Charlie also discussed fractional relaxation, which I prefer to call progressive relaxation. He took some time for questions and answers, and then came the fun!

After the evening coffee break, he told all of us to fold up the chairs and put them against the wall. Next, he had us lie down on the carpet, and then he proceeded to demonstrate how to do self-hypnosis by guiding all of us into group self-hypnosis via progressive relaxation.

The journey began, followed by pleasant relaxing and deepening suggestions, guided imagery, and post-hypnotic suggestion to be able to repeat the process. This was the only time I ever heard Charles Tebbetts use progressive relaxation as an induction; but he believed that it was the easiest way for a beginner to learn how to do self-hypnosis. Nonetheless, his self-hypnosis book contains several self-induction and deepening techniques. It also gives guidelines for suggestions used in self-hypnosis, and is written in easy-to-understand language. It contains numerous scripts and techniques, as well as some theories about hypnosis and meditation.

My own self-hypnosis book was originally self-published as *HypnoCise* in 1986. (Westwood Publishing published it a year later under a different title, *Success Through Mind Power*.) This book also presented self-hypnosis in simple language, but was slanted more for salespeople. My 1998 version, *Master the Power of Self-Hypnosis* (Sterling Publishing) was a comprehensive self-hypnosis book twice the size of the first one. After it sold out, I approached Crown House Publishing regarding my current version, and it is well suited for anyone who is interested in self-improvement! This book provides several self-inductions as well as numerous other techniques for various goals. My emphasis on the value of learning the art of self-hypnosis is evidenced by the amount I've written on that important skill.

Where do I start when teaching self-hypnosis to clients? I also teach progressive relaxation first, along with the *peaceful place meditation*. I usually incorporate stress management as well, either at the same session or at the next session; because regardless of what one does to minimize stressful situations in life, someone can always manage to push our buttons in spite of our best efforts to prevent it.

Before discussing stress coping, however, let's take a look at the peaceful place meditation and the peaceful place triggers ...

The Peaceful Place Meditation

Until 1996, I taught my clients self-hypnosis and included the stress-coping techniques without normally providing detailed explanations about establishing a "safe place" or *peaceful place*. I gave suggestions during hypnosis regarding the peaceful place, anchoring it into the mind with a *trigger* that the client can use to become more calm ... and giving ample post-hypnotic suggestions to empower the client to use his/her peaceful place trigger as desired. My experience now indicates that most people appreciate explanations about any technique that they attempt to learn for themselves. Thus, what I describe here in this chapter section is what I now do for the client AND what I tell the client will be done.

First, I remind the client of how the subconscious responded to the imaginary bucket (or magnets, etc., from the suggestibility test), emphasizing that *imagination is the language of the subconscious*. Then I explain what will happen after entering hypnosis. My wording is similar to what follows:

> **Just as the subconscious responded to what you fantasized a few minutes ago, the same can happen during the hypnotic meditation exercise ... only more so.**

> **After a few instructions to allow you to enjoy a deeper or more comfortable state of relaxation, I'll ask you to simply IMAGINE an ideal, safe or peaceful place. Your imagination is totally yours. You can do anything you wish in your imagination, and you can also be anywhere you wish as well!**

> **So when I ask you to fantasize a peaceful or pleasant place of tranquility, it is up to you to follow my simple instructions. If you try to analyze instead, or try to think of the freeway during rush-hour, you won't get your money's worth.**

I am only an artist who can say the right words, but YOU must daydream what I ask in order to maximize your benefit from this exercise.

It makes no difference whether you choose the mountains, a favorite beach, a stream, or any other place you wish. I want you to imagine sights, sounds, and feelings that are comfortable, safe, peaceful and beautiful. Remember that your subconscious does not know the difference between rehearsal and performance, as was evidenced by your response to the demonstration of the power of imagination a few minutes ago.

Also remember that the conscious mind can think MANY times faster than the spoken voice, so it makes no difference whether your conscious mind listens in or drifts and wanders, or BOTH... because you can simply DAYDREAM what I ask you to. That will help you enjoy greater benefits from this exercise.

When you really get into fantasizing your peaceful place, I'll ask you to imagine you are becoming a part of the peace that you imagine. Then I will ask you to touch your thumb to a finger that you choose to become your PEACEFUL PLACE TRIGGER.

At the same time, I'll ask you to take a deep breath and think the word RELAX while exhaling. This will anchor these actions into the subconscious so that you may use either or both as peaceful place triggers during times when your buttons get pushed.

I'll step you through this entire meditation, and then I'll give you suggestions to empower you to use the triggers and reinforce your ability by practicing this self-hypnosis exercise in the privacy of your own home or office.

Some therapists ask the client to choose and describe a peaceful place before ever starting the hypnosis, in order to use programmed imagery to describe that safe place in detail. This is optional. I normally use open-screen imagery to allow the client to create his/her place during trance, as some clients will change their minds about the place of choice after entering hypnosis. However, there are always exceptions. Be ready to be flexible to your client's needs and wishes. Also be aware that if you choose programmed imagery, you MUST know whether your client is primarily visual, auditory and/or kinesthetic ... so that you give proper imagery suggestions.

Note that a few therapists *unwisely* determine the safe place for the client. A competent hypnotherapist and psychotherapist whom I know personally used to employ programmed imagery of a beach with every client ... until he had a client scream during the induction because she had a fear of the ocean!

My friend's personal example adequately demonstrates the risk of trying to project your own ideal safe place into your client ... in other words, *fit the technique to the client rather than vice versa!* Allow your client to choose his or her ideal safe place, and then you can help anchor the triggers.

There are numerous benefits to the client for creating the peaceful place triggers ... and the peaceful place can be very helpful during hypnotherapy itself. (This can be especially true during regression therapy, as is explained in Chapter 7 of *The Art of Hypnotherapy*.) For now, I'll limit the discussion to how peaceful place triggers can help a client with both self-hypnosis and stress management.

Using the Peaceful Place Triggers

When should we use one of the peaceful place triggers?

Most of us live in a sea of stress in this modern society, and our buttons get pushed often whether we like it or not. It's normally not a question of if, but *when.*

When our buttons DO get pushed, ignoring it can hurt us. The negative emotion gets stuffed into the subconscious and comes back to haunt us later. This keeps psychotherapists, family counselors, pastoral counselors, hypnotherapists, and other professionals, etc., quite busy.

The coping skill I teach my clients is simply to *take one deep breath of air* at the times their buttons are pushed (whether or not the other peaceful place trigger is used), and then make a choice: respond now, later, or let it go.

One deep breath also becomes a trigger for staying in control and making a wise choice – and the client can use self-hypnosis to reinforce the power of that trigger. This will not solve all of life's problems, but since an ounce of prevention is worth a pound of cure, a wiser handling of emotion at the time our buttons get pushed can prevent or lessen the need for post-stress therapy.

Whenever someone does or says something that results in our having negative emotions, however, we must first accept ownership in order to deal effectively with the emotions. For example, if I say to someone, "SHE really made me mad," I just gave my power away. By changing the perception to the realization that *she sold* me the anger, and *I bought it*, I am now in control of that which I own. This perception is necessary to help me make one of the three healthy choices.

The next subsection discusses the three healthy choices as I explain to clients, and have taught repeatedly since 1984. I'll present them as though you, the reader, are my client ...

Stress Release Options – the Healthy Choices

You have three healthy options for coping with stress:

1. **Express yourself immediately but appropriately.**
    Some situations, such as your child doing something dangerous, or a sales objection during a closing interview, will require an immediate response. You may find emotion

reflected in your voice and your breath in the first example. In the second example, you may wish to take a deep breath first, and then simply express yourself calmly and confidently. In some situations, such as a customer providing a bizarre excuse to avoid paying for an item – or with your own children – you may wish to find the humorous side of the situation. Laughter can be a good release. Sometimes tears release stress; sometimes, one word spoken firmly; sometimes sarcasm; etc., etc. You decide.

2. **Express yourself later at a more appropriate time and place.**
    This option might be in your best interest if an associate at work pushes the wrong button while others are present. Some people will accept your opinion much more readily in private over coffee or tea rather than in front of peers. Furthermore, parents frequently find it more enjoyable at mealtime to insist that their children wait until after dinner to solve their arguments.

    One value from my childhood that remains with me is my father's advice: *good manners begin at home, and the table is a place of peace.* We were NOT permitted to argue at the dinner table! Neither were we punished at mealtime unless the infraction took place at the table ... in which case we were asked to leave the table. To this day I am still grateful to my father for preserving peace at mealtime.

3. **Release and let go – or, forgive.**
    If you don't choose either of the first two options, choose this one. *Forgiving does not mean condoning.* If you think someone else owes you an apology, you are the one in bondage to that belief. By freeing others from their emotional debts, you actually free yourself. Therefore, the key to forgiving is to release the other person from the apology they used to owe, and *also to forgive yourself* for buying the stress in the first place.

    You can still disapprove of the action, even though emotionally detached. (Remember this option next time someone engages in road rage and cuts into your lane! This option might literally save your life.)

Most people use other options for stress control, such as stuffing it or internalizing. The results vary from person to person: you might take it out on friends or loved ones, take it out on strangers, take it out on the same person at a later date through blowing something up all out of proportion, or take it out on yourself through sickness, or escapism, or addiction, or by becoming accident-prone. Another common option is an uncontrolled, immediate emotional expression. These options are all hazardous to our health and wealth!

In going through the healthy scenarios during self-hypnosis, remember to rehearse each of the three healthy choices. Your response to the actual stress situation in real life is like the performance – which is made much easier by proper rehearsal during self-hypnosis. You are giving yourself post-hypnotic suggestions to allow your subconscious to respond to a given signal, and *you are the one who decides when to give the signal.*

This simple technique alone has helped to increase sales commissions for many salespeople whom I've seen over the years. The reason is because emotion can be transferred from subconscious to subconscious. The client (or customer) often picks up on what the salesperson feels, whether that salesperson is stressed or feeling confident.

If you are in a sales interview and you fear losing a sale after an unexpected objection, your prospective customer may subconsciously pick up on that fear even if you use every physical sales technique in the book to cover it up. Your fear is that you might lose the sale, but your prospect's fear will be fear of making a decision – so he/she will want to "think it over" and avoid giving you the real objection.

By maintaining confidence, such confidence also comes across at a subconscious level. The prospect will be more prone to buy confidently, or have the confidence to tell you the real objection so you know where you stand. Remember that a firm "no" is better than indecision, which can drain your physical, mental, emotional and financial resources if you let it.

Practice the coping skill several times in the rehearsal room of your imagination while in a state of self-hypnosis. This helps your subconscious mind accept the desired technique at a quiet time when your emotions are not getting in the way. This is like the rehearsal, which any musician can tell you is essential before a good performance.

Doing It

Often I sell a client a copy of my newest self-hypnosis book. In some instances, I may offer a copy of this book you hold in your hands, referring to this chapter, and instruct my client on how to do self-hypnosis via progressive relaxation. Clients can find their own comfortable places, either seated, reclined or lying down – according to individual preference. (Contact lenses should be removed if necessary, and chewing gum should be discarded.)

I inform clients that the first phase of the self-hypnosis for stress management is to fantasize being in a safe, peaceful place. While imagining sights, sounds, and feelings that are pleasant and peaceful, each should then take a deep breath and think the word *"RELAX"* while exhaling. (You may also touch your thumb to a finger as an additional or alternate trigger.) The second phase is to rehearse the successful use of each of the three healthy choices in the rehearsal room of the mind. After the above, those hypnotized may awaken themselves by counting forward from one to five.

After giving the instructions, I then guide my clients into hypnosis via progressive relaxation, and guide them through the entire rehearsal. I finish with suggestions for the deep breath being a reminder that they have the power of choice, and like a muscle used becomes stronger with use, the power of choice becomes stronger with use. Just as the singer rehearses before a performance, making the performance easier, my client can rehearse his or her desired behavior in the safety of the imagination. Then, in real life, when stress buttons are pushed, that's performance time!

I conclude with a post-hypnotic suggestion for successful use of self-hypnosis, and then awaken my clients.

If you wish to make a self-hypnosis script for your client, take the progressive relaxation script from Chapter 5 of this book and change the "you" format to the first-person format; or sell him/her a copy of my self-hypnosis book, *Master the Power of Self-Hypnosis*, which has detailed instructions for how to do it.

It Only Works When it is Used

The deep breath becomes a trigger for choice – now, later, or let it go. I want it to be a reminder to all of us (myself included) that WE are owners of our own emotions, and *we have the power of choice!* Understand, too, that anyone's degree of success in coping with a stressful occurrence may vary according to the situation at hand – as well as the frequency of use of the coping technique. As a muscle is used, it becomes stronger. If it's not used, it weakens with time.

After you complete this self-hypnosis on yourself, take note of your opportunities to practice this new skill. Next time you are driving and someone turns left in front of you, take a deep breath and think the word *RELAX*. If you feel like calling him a "jerk" first, go ahead – as long as you still take the deep breath before or afterwards. Another great place to practice this skill is on the job. Suppose you are ready to go home after a hectic day at work, and you suddenly find out you have to stay late because someone else didn't finish a job. Take one deep breath, think *RELAX*, and then say and do what is appropriate.

Many of my clients have reported to me an improvement in personal self-confidence simply from mastering the art of this technique.

When I speak in public on this topic, I end my presentation with a group meditation – so that it becomes experiential for my audience. If you wish to sponsor me as a presenter for your business and/or association, contact me via e-mail at: roy@royhunter.com. If you would like hypnotic help yourself with this skill, seek a competent hypnotherapist in your area; or, if you wish, you may order my audiotape on *Stress Management* by logging onto my website (shown below). I will give a volume discount in case you wish to give or sell my tapes to your clients.

I have other tapes and training programs available, including a home study hypnosis course. If you are on the internet, check my web site at:

http://www.royhunter.com

From my home page, you can click on the pages that you wish to visit, including my CDs, books, and courses. Additionally, you may subscribe to my free e-zines.

Good luck!

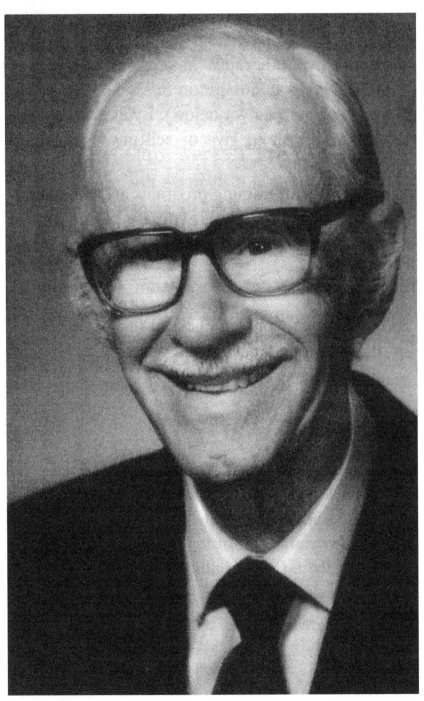

Charles Tebbetts

Chapter 11

Concepts about the Subconscious taught by Charles Tebbetts

Charles Tebbetts taught some additional concepts of the subconscious, which I present to my students at various times throughout my course. Some have already been touched on in earlier chapters where applicable; but they are organized and presented here in the same way that my mentor covered them in his "Basic Hypnosis, 101" class.

Six Functions of the Subconscious

This chapter section is summarized from the first chapter of *Self-Hypnosis and Other Mind-Expanding Techniques* (Tebbetts), and is reproduced here as on a student handout.

1. *Memory bank (like a computer)*
    The mind creates and stores records of everything that happens to us; and hypnotic regressions tap into the storehouse of memories, etc., which may be lost to the conscious mind.

    IMPORTANT: *Emotions can alter the perceptions of real events.* Do not attempt hypnotic regressions until you know how to facilitate a client abreaction and know how to avoid leading a client, as *he/she could easily mix fact with fantasy.* My students wait until halfway through the second segment of my course before learning how to facilitate a hypnotic regression.

2. *Regulates involuntary functions (heart, breathing, etc.)*
   Hypnosis can alter involuntary functions, such as slowing
   the breathing and/or heart rate, etc.; but you should avoid
   any dangerous experimentation.

   Also make certain to avoid unlicensed practice of medicine!

3. *Seat of emotions*
   When we are in a state of emotion, we are propelled toward
   what we are imagining.

   In different words, emotion is the energy dynamo – or the
   motivating power of the mind. If two emotions exist at the same
   time, the dominant one wins out over the weaker one – such
   as in the example of the ball-player WANTING to hit a home
   run, but strikes out because of his more powerful fear of
   doing so. Caught in the fear, if he imagines striking out, he is
   more prone to doing just that, as the idea of missing the ball
   is emotionally energized right into the subconscious.

   The excitement of winning can also propel an athlete into
   investing many hours of practice in order to be a winner.

4. *Seat of imagination*
   Imagination is the language of the subconscious, and imagination always seems to win out over willpower. A person
   knowing it is safe to fly still might not feel safe; and people
   who are afraid of the dark could be reacting to something
   being imagined.

5. *Controls habits*
   Nature abhors a vacuum, so new habits must replace old
   ones. Some habits are easy to eliminate; others are held
   tenaciously by the subconscious, and require hypnotherapy
   techniques to discover and remove the causes.

6. *Dynamo – directing energy that motivates us*
   The subconscious can be your master or your servant. Here
   are the words of Charles Tebbetts:

The subconscious does not think – it merely reacts!

The Five Methods of Subconscious Programming

Charles Tebbetts referred to these as the *five principles of convincing the subconscious*. They are only briefly covered here, as I incorporate some of them into my "benefits approach" for habit control and motivation – and show how that is done in Part II of this work, *The Art of Hypnotherapy*. They are the five gateways to the subconscious. I use all five in motivation mapping, presented in Chapters 15 and 16 of the hypnotherapy text.

Repetition

Repetition is the slow, hard way – but given enough times, it will work, unless there is strong subconscious resistance.

Authority figures

Those in positions of authority, be they parents, teachers, physicians, ministers, etc. – or the "authority" of proven statistics – can imprint our subconscious minds. Also, when we have an instant desire to either *obey or rebel* against a real or imagined authority, that is a subconscious reaction. This even holds true if the so-called authority is an authority-wannabe, such as a relative who pushes the "rebel" button.

Desire for identity, or identification (ego)

Identification with others, such as peer pressure, groups, parents, mentors, etc., opens the subconscious to input. Each of us has a "child inside" that wants love, belonging, acceptance and recognition – and it avoids rejection. Sometimes we tend to do undesirable things just to get attention when we need it – even if the price for that attention is high.

Hypnosis/self-hypnosis

The fact that hypnosis helps change the subconscious is why there is an entire profession dedicated to the use of hypnotherapy to help people change their lives. But unintentional uses of self-hypnosis can also imprint the subconscious, such as people smoking while tranced out in front of the T.V. set who suddenly find their ashtrays filled with cigarette remnants – but do not remember smoking that much.

Emotion

Emotions, especially intense ones, can open the subconscious to deep and long-lasting impressions. An emotionally excited person can often overcome many obstacles in achieving a goal. Also, a painful attack from a vicious dog can leave a person with a phobia of dogs for life regardless of any conscious logic, or analytical attempts to change the phobia.

Note that an easy way to remember the above gateways is with the acronym: HEARD. Each letter represents the first letter of each of the above gateways (hypnosis, emotion, authority, repetition, desire).

The Rules of the Mind

This was the very first handout I received in Edmonds. Since Charles Tebbetts gave me permission to reproduce it for all my students, I include it here – **as written in his own words**.

Some of it was previously covered where relevant, but it is organized here as my mentor wrote it. (I discuss this material in detail in a special presentation for my students.)

The words of Charles Tebbetts are printed in italics.

My additional comments are in regular type.

Rule Number One

EVERY THOUGHT OR IDEA CAUSES A PHYSICAL REACTION.

Your thoughts can affect all of the functions of your body. WORRY thoughts trigger changes in the stomach that in time can lead to ulcers. ANGER thoughts stimulate your adrenal glands and the increased adrenalin in the blood stream causes many body changes. ANXIETY and FEAR thoughts affect your pulse rate.

Ideas that have strong emotional content almost always reach the subconscious mind, because it is the feeling mind. Once accepted, these ideas continue to produce the same body reactions over and over again. In order to eliminate or change chronic negative bodily reactions we must reach the subconscious mind and change the idea responsible for the reaction. This is easily done with self-hypnosis and autosuggestion.

Charles Tebbetts believed that the mind could make you sick or keep you well. For example, he believed that a person could easily produce a headache just by imagining one. He also demonstrated the ultimate benefit of self-hypnosis when a stroke totally paralyzed him and left him unable to talk. Through self-hypnosis, he recovered – and continued to teach hypnotherapy for many years afterward.

Rule Number Two

WHAT'S EXPECTED TENDS TO BE REALIZED.

The brain and the nervous system respond only to mental images. It does not matter if the image is self-induced or from the external world. The mental image formed becomes the blueprint, and the subconscious mind uses every means at its disposal to carry out the plan. Worrying is a form of programming a picture of what we don't want. But the subconscious mind acts to fulfill the pictured situation. "THE THINGS THAT I HAVE FEARED HAVE COME UPON ME."

Many persons suffer from chronic anxiety, which is simply a subconscious mental expectancy that something terrible will happen. On the other hand, we all know people who seem to have the "magic" touch. Life seems to shower them with blessings for no apparent reason, and so we call them "lucky." What seems to be luck is in reality POSITIVE MENTAL EXPECTANCY, a strong belief that success is deserved. "WE BECOME WHAT WE THINK ABOUT."

Physical health is largely dependent upon our mental expectancy. Physicians recognize that if a patient expects to remain sick, lame, paralyzed, helpless, even to die, the expected condition tends to be realized. Here is where self-hypnosis can become the tool to remove despondency and negative attitudes and bring about a hopeful positive expectancy – the expectancy of health, strength and well-being, which then tends to be realized.

This is also called the law of expectancy (as previously mentioned in Chapter 8). He told my class about a man who died while being bathed by a nurse, because he had a total expectation that if he were ever bathed, it would be fatal. Although the nurse scoffed at this man's belief and bathed him over his screaming protests, his expectation still produced a deadly result. Mr. Tebbetts wrote about this case in the first chapter of *Self-Hypnosis and Other Mind-Expanding Techniques*.

In order for a client to achieve a permanent success even with hypnosis, the expectation must somehow become positive for lasting success; otherwise, even if a smoker sees the best hypnotherapist in the world, failure may devour initial success. If he or she *expects* to backslide, it is only a matter of time before the expectation will be realized. When Charles Tebbetts used self-hypnosis to recover from his stroke, his recovery was permanent until the day of his death.

Rule Number Three

IMAGINATION IS MORE POWERFUL THAN KNOWLEDGE WHEN DEALING WITH THE MIND.

This is an important rule to remember when using self-hypnosis. REASON IS EASILY OVERRULED BY IMAGINATION. This is why some persons blindly rush into some unreasonable act or situation. Violent crimes based upon jealousy are almost always caused by an over-active imagination. Most of us feel superior to those who lose their savings to confidence men, or blindly follow a demagogue such as Hitler or are sold worthless stocks. We can easily see that such people have allowed the imagination to overcome the reason. But we are often blind to our own superstitions, prejudices, and unreasonable beliefs. Any idea accompanied by a strong emotion such as anger, hatred, love, or political and religious beliefs usually cannot be modified through the use of reason. In using self-hypnosis we can form images in the subconscious mind which is the feeling mind, and can remove, alter or amend the old ideas.

This is also called the law of conflict. Stated another way, WHENEVER IMAGINATION AND LOGIC ARE IN CONFLICT, IMAGINATION USUALLY WINS.

To explain this concept easily to a group of people, I often ask, "If a plank three feet wide and fifty feet long were placed one inch off the ground, and someone offered to give you ten thousand dollars for walking its length without stepping off – and it was a clear day with no breeze – how many of you have total confidence that you would successfully do so?" Now try putting the same plank between the top of two skyscrapers and watch what happens to your confidence. The only major difference is the penalty for stepping off! However, the power of imagination would make it dangerous even for me to walk across the plank in those circumstances – because my imagination would work overtime imagining the deadly drop to the pavement below.

Always remember that *imagination is the language of the subconscious.*

I believe it is important to help my clients imagine total success before I bring them out of hypnosis – and I also suggest that they vividly remember the success that they have imagined, as the mind often responds to what we imagine.

Rule Number Four

OPPOSING IDEAS CANNOT BE HELD AT ONE AND THE SAME TIME.

This does not mean more than one idea cannot be remembered or harbored in your memory, but it refers to the conscious mind recognizing an idea. Many people try to hold opposing ideas simultaneously. A man might believe in honesty and expect his children to be honest, and all the while be engaging daily in slightly dishonest business practices. He may try to justify by saying: "All of my competitors do it, it's an accepted practice." However, he cannot escape the conflict and its effect upon his nervous system that is caused by trying to hold opposing ideas within himself.

When I was in college, my summer employer one year was a deacon in the Baptist church who prided himself on being an honest family man. His wife – who was one of my aunts – told me that her husband never swore, never drank, and that he always told the truth even when it hurt. But within one hour on the job, I heard more profanity than I normally heard in a month. Furthermore, dishonest business practices (that reflected total greed) became a disillusioning shock, which he claimed to be "common business practice." I might add that, true to what Charles Tebbetts said concerning this rule of the mind, my uncle could not handle the stress of his double standard. He died young of a heart attack.

Rule Number Five

ONCE AN IDEA HAS BEEN ACCEPTED BY THE SUBCON-SCIOUS MIND, IT REMAINS UNTIL IT IS REPLACED BY ANOTHER IDEA. The companion rule to this is: THE LONGER THE IDEA REMAINS, THE MORE OPPOSITION THERE IS TO REPLACING IT WITH A NEW IDEA.

Once an idea has been accepted, it tends to remain. The longer it is held, the more it tends to become a fixed habit of thinking. This is how habits of action are formed, both good and bad. First there is the thought and then the action. We have habits of thinking as well as habits of action, but the thought or idea always comes first. Hence it is obvious if we wish to change actions we must begin by changing thoughts. We accept as true certain facts. For example, we accept as true that the sun rises in the east and sets in the west and we accept this even though the day may be cloudy and we cannot see the sun. This is an instance of a correct fact conception which governs our actions under normal conditions. However, we have many thought habits which are not correct and yet are fixed in the mind. Some people believe that at critical times they must have a drink of whiskey or a tranquilizer to steady their nerves so that they can perform effectively. This is not correct but the idea is there, and is a fixed habit of thought. There will be opposition to replacing it with a correct idea.

Now in advancing these rules, we are speaking of fixed ideas, not just idle thoughts or passing fancies. We need to alter fixed ideas or to use them. No matter how fixed the ideas may be or how long they have remained they can be changed with either or both self-hypnosis and autosuggestion.

A child attacked by a vicious dog may get the idea that dogs are dangerous. If that idea persists, then the phobia will become more sensitized every time a dog growls or barks at that child. Also, a person going up and down like a yo-yo with one diet after another can also become sensitized to the idea of failing at weight reduction; thus it becomes increasingly more difficult to believe in the ability ever to maintain control over his/her weight.

Rule Number Six

AN EMOTIONALLY INDUCED SYMPTOM TENDS TO CAUSE ORGANIC CHANGE IF PERSISTED IN LONG ENOUGH.

It has been acknowledged by many reputable medical men that more than seventy percent of human ailments are functional rather than organic. This means that the function of an organ or other part of the body has been disturbed by the reaction of the nervous system to negative ideas held in the subconscious mind. We do not mean to imply that every person who complains of an ailment is emotionally ill or neurotic. There are diseases caused by germs, parasites, virus, and other things attacking the human body. However, we are a mind in a body and the two cannot be separated. Therefore, if you continue to fear ill health, constantly talk about your "nervous stomach" or "tension headaches," in time organic changes must occur.

Psychosomatic illness is a fact; and most of us realize that prolonged stress can have a negative impact on our health.

Rule Number Seven

EACH SUGGESTION ACTED UPON CREATES LESS OPPOSITION TO SUCCESSIVE SUGGESTION.

A mental trend is easier to follow the longer it lasts unbroken. Once a habit is formed it becomes easier to follow and more difficult to break.

*In other words once a self-suggestion has been accepted by your
subconscious mind, it becomes easier for additional suggestions to
be accepted and acted upon. That is why when you are just beginning with self-hypnosis and autosuggestion we suggest you start
with simple suggestions. You can suggest that you feel a tingling
sensation or a warm and pleasant feeling. When these have been
followed you can move on to more complicated suggestions. You
should begin now with the suggestion that you will automatically
awaken from self-hypnosis in ten minutes.*

This can also be called the rule of compound suggestion, briefly
mentioned in Chapter 8.

Stage hypnotists frequently use compound suggestion for deepening the trance when using hypnosis for entertainment, often adding greater expectancy for entertaining responses to post-hypnotic
suggestion at the end of the show. This same principle can be used
to build expectation so that the therapeutic post-hypnotic suggestions to change a habit will become more effective.

Rule Number Eight

WHEN DEALING WITH THE SUBCONSCIOUS MIND
AND ITS FUNCTIONS, THE GREATER THE CONSCIOUS
EFFORT, THE LESS THE SUBCONSCIOUS RESPONSE.

*This proves why "will-power" doesn't really exist! If you have
insomnia you've learned "the harder you try to go to sleep, the
more wide awake you become." The rule is when dealing with the
subconscious mind, TAKE IT EASY. This means you must work
to develop a positive mental expectancy that your problem can
be and will be solved. As your faith in your subconscious mind
increases you learn to "let it happen" rather than trying to "force
it to happen."*

I frequently tell my clients that trying to use "willpower" or self-discipline to quit smoking often comes across to the subconscious just

like a high pressure salesman trying to force us to buy something we don't want.

The subconscious can be persuaded, but it cannot be forced without resistance. Hypnotherapy's primary claim to fame is in helping clients achieve goals that subconscious resistance prevents them from achieving on their own.

Many hypnotherapists talk about "facilitating" a session. Personally, I like this term because the very word implies that we are making something easy, so that it requires less effort. Let's use appropriate ethical and considerate hypnotic techniques to help the client succeed as easily as possible.

So... WHERE DO WE GO FROM HERE?

My own professional experience resulted in updates in what I presented in this chapter as well as throughout this entire book.

If you purchased this book simply because you are curious about hypnosis, you should now know more about hypnosis than 90 to 95 percent of the general public. If you are a student of hypnosis OR a professional, hopefully this book will prove to be a great benefit in helping you enhance both your knowledge and your confidence in the art of hypnosis.

By now the serious student of hypnosis should have enough information to help learn the art of hypnosis and master basic techniques.

If you are applying what I teach in this book, you should be able to accomplish the following: to prepare a client for entering hypnosis; to guide a willing client into the hypnosis (alpha) state; to deepen appropriately and estimate trance depth; to give suggestions that will help validate the trance state in the mind of your client; to successfully give properly structured suggestions; to manage the typical non-therapeutic aspects of hypnosis; to awaken your client comfortably and completely; to have a grasp of hypnosis ethics and potential pitfalls; to teach and practice the peaceful place meditation (and a self-hypnosis technique for stress management); and to have a basic understanding of the rules of the mind.

When you develop confidence and competence in these areas – and are willing to practice hypnosis with integrity and with a sincere desire to help your clients – you are ready to learn hypnotherapy techniques.

My students have gone through the information presented in these eleven chapters by the time they finish the first three months of my nine-month hypnotherapy course. In addition to weekly classes, they attend an all-day workshop, read a book about hypnosis or hypnotherapy, write a review (and provide other students with copies); and they must complete twenty-four non-therapeutic hypnosis practice sessions – mostly with other students. Other instructors teaching my course have similar requirements.

Some students become anxious to get past the basics and into the second quarter; but most seem to appreciate the time spent in basic training – as evidenced repeatedly by class evaluations from well-educated professionals who have taken my course. Understanding their quest for information, however, I frequently *preview* the remainder of my course through a brief discussion of hypnotherapy. If time permits, I also provide an introduction to the legendary parts therapy taught and used by Charles Tebbetts.

At the request of the organization that published the first edition of this book, I have also done likewise for you, the reader, by adding another chapter to this text. Even at the dawn of the new millennium, it seems appropriate to retain and update that chapter for my Millennium Edition of *The Art of Hypnosis*.

Thank you for continuing your journey with me this far ...

Chapter 12

Introducing the Art of Hypnotherapy

As mentioned at the conclusion of the last chapter, my students usually get a preview of the art of hypnotherapy before completing Beginning Hypnosis. So now I'll preview *The Art of Hypnotherapy* (with a preface by Joyce Tebbetts), also available from Crown House Publishing. This chapter overviews that book (formerly Parts II & III of the Charles Tebbetts Hypnotism Training Course), and previews my mentor's legendary *parts therapy*.

Here's the Table of Contents ...

I'll again remind the reader that *all hypnotherapy employs the use of hypnosis; but not all hypnosis is hypnotherapy.*

So... Just What is Hypnotherapy?

Let's begin with an overview of the first chapter, which looks at what Mr. Tebbetts presented on the third page of *Miracles on Demand* (2nd edition):

> *Hypnotherapy works on the principle that most maladaptive behavior is the result of inappropriate adjustive responses chosen to attain infantile needs which are no longer necessary to an adult. The role of the hypno-therapist is usually to shift the client's interpretation of her environment from that necessary to a child to that appropriate to an adult.*

He goes on to point out that while traditional therapies deal with symptoms on a cognitive or intellectual level (dealing with the conscious mind), hypnotherapy bypasses the critical factor of the conscious analyzing mind and goes right to the subconscious – which is the seat of the emotions as well as the storehouse of memories. To effectively do this requires a working knowledge of a variety of effective hypnotherapy techniques as well as both confidence and competence with the art of hypnosis – not only in guiding a client into hypnosis, but also in knowing how to keep him/her deep enough to obtain results.

Now let's consider the difference between hypnosis and hypno-therapy, as my own opinion has changed since the first edition of this book...

For 15 years I taught that one could define hypnotherapy as: *the use of hypnosis or any hypnotic technique to enhance goal achievement, to enhance motivation or change, to enhance personal or spiritual growth, and/or to release clients of problems and the causes of problems.*

I believed that this simplified definition was true whether the use for hypnotherapy was medical or non-medical, as medical symptoms can also be called problems – whether removed by a physician directly, or by a trained hypnotherapist working under a physician's referral or direct supervision.

Events of the late 1990s have prompted me to update my definition of hypnotherapy because many *hypnotists* claim to be hypnotherapists after only three to five days of training, including some who believe that a background in mental health counseling is a substitute for competent training in the art of hypnotherapy. They might learn a few induction techniques, and blend them with a script book ... in hopes that post-hypnotic suggestion alone can help people overcome problems. While this works for some of the people some of the time, it does NOT work for all the people all the time, even when accompanied by counseling.

Hypnotist or Hypnotherapist?

Those who attempt to help people by suggestion alone (and have often taken only a short 3-day or 5-day training program) should, in my professional opinion, use the title of "Certified Hypnotist" rather than promoting themselves as a "Certified Hypnotherapist." Let's explore this further ...

A hypnotist can give positive suggestions, and use scripts to help people who need motivation – often with profound results ... but what about those who resist suggestion?

Whenever subconscious resistance inhibits a client's ability to respond to suggestion and imagery, *hypnotherapy* is required to help the subconscious to discover and release the cause(s) of the problem. The competent hypnotherapist knows how to accomplish this, but the hypnotist all-too-often tells the client something like, "You are resisting, so you probably aren't ready for hypnosis yet."

In short, the hypnotist simply gives many suggestions and hopes for results, while the hypnotherapist knows how to solicit the subconscious to reveal the cause(s) in order to facilitate release and relearning ... and resolve problems.

Many people who claim to be a *Certified Hypnotherapist* could, in my opinion, more accurately be called a *Certified Hypnotist* or "consulting hypnotist" because they use only the first hypnotherapy step described in the next chapter section rather than all four. In other words, they often rely on suggestion alone to help people change ... and then may actually blame the client if he/she fails to achieve the stated goal! If and when the major recognized hypnosis associations realize this, I believe that it will be a GREAT benefit to the credibility of the hypnotherapy profession!

Indeed, this is still a gray area; but let me ask YOU, the reader, an important question: if you desired hypnotherapy, would you trust a hypnotist who spent only a few days in training (even if he or she was a psychotherapist), or would you rather invest your time and money with someone who invested several months in training? I'll choose the latter, regardless of whether or not that person holds a graduate degree.

If hypnotherapy is needed rather than simply motivation, the competently trained hypnotherapist is far more able to help you. However, if all you need is help with motivation, then you might enjoy success with either a hypnotist or a hypnotherapist.

It is my hope (and prayer) that our recognized hypnosis associations will soon find a way to UNITE and create uniform standards to define the qualifications of a "Certified Hypnotist" and a "Certified Hypnotherapist." Truly I believe this will benefit both the profession AND the general public.

How Can Hypnotherapy Resolve Problems?

Now let's briefly overview hypnotherapy for problem resolution. According to my late mentor, there are four basic steps to resolving a client's problem and/or changing an undesired habit. He taught them in class, and discussed them in both editions of *Miracles on Demand*. These are summarized in Chapter 3 of my next book, and woven in throughout the rest of that text; so I'll briefly discuss them here. I consider them to be the foundation of client-centered hypnotherapy.

1.   **Suggestion and Imagery:** Simply use *direct or indirect sugges-tion* during hypnosis, and/or imagery. This may be sufficient only if the *motivating desire is strong,* unless the problem stems from a traumatic experience. Simply hypnotizing someone and relying on the power of suggestion alone is what Charles Tebbetts called "Band-Aid therapy." It may or may not make a difference; and the changes may only be temporary – as sometimes happened with the 19th century pioneers of hypnosis who relied totally on prestige suggestion alone. Sometimes simply changing the response to a trigger can help a client replace one habit with another, such as one deep breath to replace a cigarette. Various imagery techniques can also be employed to enable the client to imagine fulfillment of his/her goal as well as the desired accompanying benefits of success, including those employed in the *benefits approach* (Chapter 4). A competent hypnotist can help someone who only needs this first step; thus many hypnotists can brag about profound results and show convincing testimonial letters from satisfied clients. But what happens when there is subconscious resistance?

2.   **Discover the cause:** Use one (or more) of many various hyp-notherapy techniques to *discover the cause* of a problem. This is necessary when the first step is not enough to help a client achieve success! The cause, or memory, is provoked – along with accompanying feelings – which the client is allowed (but not forced) to feel. This is easily accomplished while a client is in the state of hypnosis; but this step should only be employed when you know how to competently facilitate client abreactions. Parts therapy, regression therapy, and/or numerous other techniques can be used for this step as well as for the next two steps. Also we should note that many techniques designed to discover (or uncover) the cause of a problem may result in a hypnotic regression. Even indirect suggestion scripts designed to make this process happen at a subconscious level could still result in client abreactions.

Also note that some causes of problems may be *present* unresolved issues rather than past ones (and may require other help besides hypnosis). Note that an entire chapter of *The Art of Hypnotherapy* (Chapter 6) is devoted to various techniques taught by Charles Tebbetts to help uncover causes of subconscious resistance; and Chapter 7 is devoted exclusively to hypnotic regressions. (My students do NOT attempt hypnotic regressions until they are four months into their training, and understand the important difference between leading and guiding.)

3. **Release:** *Facilitate release* from the cause of the problem. In order to pave the way for release, we must first *establish the relationship* of the cause of the problem at both an emotional and logical level. Release of a client's present unresolved issue may require other professional help besides hypnosis. Also, such release may either be from actual memories of real past events, whether conscious or repressed, or from *perceptions* of events which may have been altered by the subconscious through the years. If those past perceptions are *released and/or forgiven,* it normally will NOT be necessary to wade through all past perceptions to sort out the real memories from the distorted or false memories. This process is detailed in the regression chapter of *The Art of Hypnotherapy,* along with some very important information concerning the difference between guiding and leading.

    Release of relevant past event(s) or perceptions can usually be accomplished through forgiveness or release. Also, since we cannot hope for a better past, we might as well *forgive* – and put our energies into building a better present and future! (Forgiving does not mean condoning.) Besides facilitating release, competently facilitated hypnotic regression usually guides the client right into the next step.

4. **Subconscious relearning:** Find a way to *facilitate subconscious or emotional relearning* which will allow the client to make future decisions unencumbered by the formerly repressed material and/or negative beliefs. Mr. Tebbetts taught a variety of techniques to help accomplish this. Some of the

various techniques taught by my mentor to facilitate both release and relearning include parts therapy, regression therapy, Gestalt therapy, verbalizing, open screen imagery, indirect guided imagery, implosive desensitization, systematic desensitization, object projection, and more. *Several* chapters of *The Art of Hypnotherapy* explain these very effective client-centered techniques.

Note that when the first step is insufficient, then the first step becomes the last step.

Are All These Steps Necessary?

The answer varies from person to person, because each client is different and has his/her unique personality. Even Charles Tebbetts admitted that the first step was sometimes sufficient for motivation and some habit changes – and was *frequently* sufficient to help people quit smoking or for other motivation goals.

My own *benefits approach* is an effective way to strengthen the motivating desires in a positive way through the use of hypnotic *progression* – which often gets results with little or no need of regressions or parts therapy, thus utilizing only the first step. Remember, however, that many people will require all four steps – and if you are not trained in hypnotic regressions, nor unless you understand the handling of abreactions, then be prepared to *refer some of your clients* to those who are qualified and trained in techniques that take a client through the last three steps.

Some people, especially facilitators of large groups, often use aversion techniques, thus skipping the last three steps. For example, smokers are shown graphic pictures of diseased lungs, etc., and then told in hypnosis to visualize disease. This leaves one to wonder what potential consequences might happen to the person still smoking if the mind indulges in constant negative images. To all who do group sessions – please *REFER your participants for the necessary appropriate follow-up* and create a win/win for all. Please help support the local hypnotherapists.

Now let's wrap up my comments about the four steps.

These steps form the four cornerstones for building a solid foundation of success – for any therapeutic modality you use to help your client achieve ideal empowerment. These important steps are the four main objectives of successful hypnotherapy, regardless of which tools you use.

Just knowing what the steps are is not nearly as important as knowing how to *competently* use any technique to facilitate client success! That is especially true of the parts therapy that helped make Charles Tebbetts become a living legend during his lifetime. It is the most complex hypnotic tool available as the new millennium dawns, yet it is profoundly effective when used properly – so let's preview it now.

Preview of Parts Therapy

Before I provide an overview of parts therapy (also called *ego state* therapy), I must precede this chapter section with a warning! *Please do NOT use parts therapy unless or until you have received competent training in BOTH regression therapy and parts therapy.*

My mentor believed that we all have various aspects of the personality, which he called *ego parts*. In the hypnotic state, one may actually call out these various "parts" of the personality and facilitate dialogue.

Wise and appropriate use of parts therapy can help the client with inner conflicts come to internal resolution – but it is extremely important that such dialogue be *totally client-centered* rather than therapist-directed or ego-centered! It's important that the therapist *avoids* forming preconceived opinions about the cause(s) of the problem, as the opinions could be projected into the client and taint the trance. (Often this is more difficult for the trained diagnostician than it is for the hypnotherapist who does not diagnose!) The subconscious may come up with an entirely different cause than the one that may be arrived at by either client or therapist through conscious discussion prior to hypnosis. It is very important for the facilitator to act like a mediator, staying objective.

An effective parts therapy session incorporates at least three (and often all four) of the hypnotherapeutic steps to facilitate change, involving the entire hypnotherapeutic process. I devoted a very lengthy chapter to it in my next text.

Examples of Clients with Successful Parts Therapy

One of the most profound examples of a successful client of parts therapy is a man I know personally who experienced a session with Charles Tebbetts in the late 1980s.

His real name is Scott, and he lives near Seattle. He had a medical referral to see Charlie for epilepsy. Scott told me that he was *determined* to make a change (and his own commitment to making a change was very important!), yet he felt that traditional therapy was not helping him. Just one session of parts therapy helped him discover a great deal about himself. His subconscious told him why the subconscious originally produced epilepsy; but when that cause was released, the subconscious then gave a second reason for keeping it as an adult: *drinking*. That part of him wanting to drink was told by another part that if he gave up drinking, he could be released from epilepsy. I obtained a copy of the therapy session on videotape, along with his permission to discuss his case in my advanced text. I show this session to my own students during the Advanced Hypnotherapy segment of my course. Chapter 12 of *The Art of Hypnotherapy* contains most of the actual script from the session itself. Not only has Scott remained sober (as of the second edition of this book), he has not had even one seizure in a decade since his session! (You can purchase this DVD online if you wish by going to my website at www.royhunter.com and clicking on products.)

Charles Tebbetts wrote about numerous case histories with parts therapy in his book, *Miracles on Demand* – which I hope comes back into print again sometime. All of the case histories he wrote about were documented on videotape. Even though some of them have become lost over the years, I still have a few recordings in my possession – which Charlie personally gave to me while he was still living. Some are shown in my classroom.

Here are some of my own client successes. (The names are changed to protect client confidentiality.)

Ron, an overweight client who was self-employed, had an inner child that felt he was working too hard – so excess junk food was his recreation until he agreed to balance his life by taking more time for personal fun and recreation.

Betty, an overweight counselor/therapist, had a part (like Ron did) making her fat by overeating in order to punish her for working too many hours and not taking time for herself.

Linda, a smoker, failed to respond to my usual benefits approach. One part wanted to live long and prosper, while another part felt compelled to make a statement of rebellion against society manipulating her into quitting. This same part really wanted choice – so when another part of her convinced her that she was actually being manipulated into smoking by other people's prejudice, she realized that she was giving her power of choice away every time she lit up!

Ted, an insurance salesman afraid of rejection, was in conflict with his desire to reach sales quota – because his father imprinted him with the belief that successful salespeople are dishonest. This resulted in regression therapy.

Joan was a workaholic professional woman who lacked confidence and felt compelled to "prove her worth in a man's world" simply because a part of her was angry at her father for wishing she had been a boy. A more spiritual part told her to forgive Dad and get on with her own life.

Randy was a hypnotherapist who felt unworthy to be in this profession. He had a perfectionist part that felt nothing was good enough unless it was done perfectly.

Bill was a realtor who kept getting bogged down with too much paperwork even in prospecting habits, because as a child he had been told repeatedly, "Don't do a job unless you do it right!" His subconscious kept making him work twice as hard as necessary until his parts came to terms of agreement.

Get trained first

Effectively facilitated, parts therapy is one of the most profound techniques available for facilitating change. But even if you are already a certified hypnotherapist, please *do not attempt parts therapy until you have been trained in all the steps!* Skilled use of parts therapy incorporates other hypnotherapy techniques and/or results in spontaneous hypnotic regressions. Mistakes made by those who shortcut proper training can leave a client confused, disoriented, or worse. For example, simply forgetting to explain the concept properly to a client in advance could leave him/her fearing multiple personalities! Or if the therapist makes a part angry by trying to force it to change, the client could actually get worse – and experience has proven that people with advanced degrees are not immune to making such mistakes.

This chapter was meant simply to *introduce* you to the concept of parts therapy – *not* to make you an expert. Again, I urge you to get actual training before using it; or, at the *very least*, read *The Art of Hypnotherapy* first.

As my schedule permits, I will make myself available to those who wish "hands-on" training of all or part of my course. Contact me directly if interested at (253) 927-8888 or e-mail me at: roy@ royhunter.com.

If you desire additional information, read the official alt.hypnosis FAQ on my website at the following URL: *http://www.royhunter. com/hypnofaq.htm.*

Please respect the value of my time if you e-mail me for advice. I have received e-mails from both the general public and from professionals all over the world asking me for free professional advice. While I would like to provide personal replies to all who wish it, my time simply does not permit me to give lengthy answers to everyone ... so please be prepared to compensate me for any ongoing e-mail correspondence.

In Conclusion

If you are already a trained and certified hypnotherapist, I hope your time invested in reading this information I teach in Basic Hypnosis still proves to be a worthy investment for both you and your clients. Hopefully you've learned a few new techniques and/or a better way of perceiving hypnosis. Perhaps this book can be an easy-reading reference guide.

If you are a hypnosis student, I strongly recommend that you seek "hands-on" training from a certified hypnotherapy instructor who is familiar with what is presented in this book, and whose course is credentialed by at least one national hypnosis association. Avoid self-certifying instructors whose only certification is with an association where they have a vested interest. This skill is too important for "quick-fix" training by people only in it for quick profit. If this country were not littered with so many short-cut hypnosis programs, I would not have to emphasize this so much.

Also, please DO NOT assume that you can adequately master an art just by reading about it! Be willing to allow an experienced hypnotherapy instructor to critique you as you demonstrate your hypnotic skills.

Based on your desired future uses of hypnosis as well as your own educational background, you may decide whether to seek training by those within the scientific community – or by those of us dedicated to the full-time profession of hypnotherapy, emphasizing its non-medical uses. Hopefully this book can help you make that choice if you have not already done so; and you can use my book as a reference regardless of your choice.

So now your *journey has just begun.*

The *Art of Hypnotherapy* teaches a logical multi-modality approach to hypnotherapy. You'll learn how to help clients sell success to their subconscious minds. You'll explore various client-centered techniques mastered and taught by my late friend and mentor, Charles Tebbetts, and updated by my professional experience – techniques to help discover and release subconscious resistance to success, and to help your clients become more self-empowered to achieve their goals, in order to *believe in their success!*

My next book closes with some comments and personal opinions about our profession's ongoing mission. It is written to help you learn and master the *art of hypnotherapy.*

The journey has just begun ...

Glossary

Common Hypnosis Terms
& Abbreviations

abreaction: emotional discharge, usually due to remembering past pain

affirmations: positive statements designed to change subconscious programming

age regression: guiding a hypnotized person backwards in time by his/her age
WARNING: Only those trained in regression therapy should do this!

alpha: a state of the mind where brainwave activity slows down to a range of from 7–14 cycles per second, during which we experience hypnosis, and which we pass through on the way to and from sleep daily

altered consciousness: synonymous with alpha; terminology used to refer to the state of mind we experience during hypnosis, meditation, or any form of trance

anchoring: establishing a trigger which, when activated, will trigger certain responses; this happens randomly in life, but can be suggested during hypnosis (see also triggers)

aversion suggestion: suggestions given that emphasize negative aspects of a habit, such as finding smoke to smell horrible and/or make someone sick

awakening: the act of bringing a person up out of trance and into full conscious awareness

beta: that state of mind we are in during most of our waking hours, the thinking mode

deepening: in hypnosis, this refers to attaining a more profound trance state

delta: that state of mind we enter during deep sleep, total unconsciousness

direct suggestion: suggestions given as commands ("take a deep breath")

expectancy: having expectations of a certain outcome

eye fixation: induction involving staring at an object

false memories: fantasies that are experienced during a mishandled regression which are believed to be repressed memories rather than fantasies

FMS: abbreviation for False Memory Syndrome (having false memories)

Gestalt therapy: involves role-playing (often used for release)

HypnoCise: a word coined by the FAQ author to describe the combination of imagery, meditation, self-hypnosis and properly constructed affirmations

hypnosis: a trance state which is guided by someone or something other than the person experiencing the trance (there are numerous definitions by different experts)

hypnotherapist: a trained professional who uses hypnosis to help people with self-improvement and/or for therapeutic purposes

hypnotherapy: the use of hypnosis for self-improvement and/or for therapeutic purposes

hypnotist: anyone who guides another person into hypnosis

ideomotor responding: having client answer questions via finger movement

imagery: using the imagination to fantasize or remember events

indirect suggestion: permissive suggestions ("you can take a deep breath whenever you wish to relax")

induction: a technique that guides (induces) a person into a hypnotic state

initial sensitizing event: an emotional event that is the ORIGIN of a problem, creating a sensitivity to feelings; such as claustrophobia being traced back to being locked in a closet at age 3

ISE: abbreviation for Initial Sensitizing Event

NLP: abbreviation for Neuro-Linguistic Programming, a modality of change that evolved from the teachings of Milton Erickson

NS: abbreviation for Non-Smoking programs

old tapes: a term frequently used to describe memories that are replayed in the imagination in a manner that may influence our behavior and/or attitudes

original sensitizing event: alternate name for initial sensitizing event

parts therapy: a complex hypnotic technique where the therapist talks with various parts of the mind, such as the inner child and inner adult

WARNING: Only those trained in parts therapy should use it!

past life therapy: regression into real or imagined past life

PLR: abbreviation for Past Life Regression

PLT: abbreviation for Past Life Therapy (PLR is used more often)

post-hypnotic suggestion: a suggestion given during the trance state which is acted upon after emerging from the trance state

PR: abbreviation for Progressive Relaxation

progressive relaxation: a type of induction involving the progressive relaxation of various parts of the body

PT: abbreviation for Parts Therapy

rapport: a comfortable feeling between client and hypnotist resulting in a level of trust, resulting in greater ability to respond to suggestion

reframing: using the imagination to imagine a different outcome of a past event, such as combining Gestalt therapy with regression therapy to facilitate release; also used in NLP with guided imagery

regression: going back in time during trance to remember past events, and replaying them in the imagination, often with accompanying emotions

self-hypnosis: a self-induced trance state

stage hypnosis: the public use of hypnosis purely for entertainment purposes

subconscious: that part of our mind which is the seat of imagination, emotion, artistic abilities (and other skills), and which takes care of numerous functions without our conscious awareness, such as automatic functions of our organs, etc.

subjects (of hypnosis): the term used by many to describe a person who is in hypnosis (NOTE: the word "client" is used with increasing frequency by hypnotherapists)

systematic desensitization: the use of programmed imagery in a systematic way to help desensitize someone from an anxiety or phobia

theta: that state of mind we are in while dreaming time distortion: the term for a unique phenomenon where we lose conscious awareness of how much time has passed (examples: 5 minutes can seem like 20 minutes, or vice versa)

triggers: something seen, heard, felt, etc., which "triggers" a response, urge, memory, or emotion, etc., such as turning the key in the car might "trigger" a smoker to light up a cigarette
WT: abbreviation for WeighT
zzz: sleeeeeeeeep (go waaaaay down deep!)
*The glossary is taken from the one that I prepared for the official FAQ "alt.hypnosis" worldwide internet newsgroup. (Note: FAQ is an acronym for Frequently Asked Questions.) The current version of the FAQ is stored at my website at the following URL: www. royhunter.com. Follow the link to the FAQ. Also, I have self-help and training materials available that can be purchased online.

Bibliography

Counseling Hypnotherapy: The Synergism of Psychotherapy and Hypnotherapy (Charles J. Francis, M.A., A.C.H.) National Guild of Hypnotists
Experiencing Hypnosis (Erickson and Rossi) Irvington Publishing, 1981
General Techniques of Hypnotism (Andre Weitzenhoffer, PhD) Out of print
Hypnosis and Hypnotherapy (Helmut W. A. Karle) Out of print
Hypnosis Induction Technics (Myron Teitelbaum, M.D., J.D.) Charles C. Thomas Publishing Ltd., 1969
Hypnosis: The Cognitive-Behavioral Perspective (Nicholas Spanos and John Chaves) Prometheus Books, 1989
Hypnosis: The Induction of Conviction (John C. Hughes, D.C.) National Guild of Hypnotists
Hypnosis: Understanding How It Can Work for You (Sean Kelly, PhD; Reid Kelly, A.C.S.W.) Out of print
Hypnotherapy (Dave Elman) Westwood Publishing, 1984
Hypnotic Inductions & Prescriptions (Arthur E. Winkler, PhD) St. John's University
Hypnotic Investigation of Psychodynamic Processes (Milton H. Erickson, M.D.; ed. by Ernest Rossi, PhD) Irvington Publishing, 1980
Hypnotic Realities (Erickson and Rossi) Irvington Publishing, 1976
Hypnotism Today (LeCron and Bordeaux) Out of print
Love, Medicine & Miracles (Bernie S. Siegel, M.D.) Harperperennial Library, 1990
Mesmerism and the End of Enlightenment in France (Robert Darnton) Harvard University Press, 1986
Miracles on Demand (Charles Tebbetts, 2nd edition) Out of print
Mosby Medical Encyclopedia (1992 edition)
Psychosemantic Parenthetics (James F. Russell, PhD) Out of print
Self-Hypnotism (Leslie M. LeCron, PhD) Out of print
Self-Hypnosis and Other Mind-Expanding Techniques (Charles Tebbetts, 3rd edition) 1st ed. available from Westwood Publishing, 1977
Stress and the Art of Biofeedback (Barbara B. Brown) Out of print
The Wisdom of Milton H. Erickson (Ronald A. Havens) Irvington Publishing, 1989
The Young Freud: The Origins of Psychoanalysis in Late Nineteenth-Century Viennese Culture (Billa Zanuso) Out of print
NOTE: If you are a researcher who wishes to read the books that are out of print, check with your local library. Some libraries might still carry the books that are out of print.

Index

NOTE: Chapters are in *bold italics*.

Do you have the second volume yet?

The Art of Hypnotherapy
by C. Roy Hunter, M.S., FAPHP
with Preface by Joyce Tebbetts

This important second volume has been praised by many professionals.

You may order from the author's website:
http://www.royhunter.com/hypnosis_books.htm

Or you may order directly from the publisher:
http://www.crownhousepublishing.com